Dana Carpender

PALEO/ PRIMAL

IN 5 INGREDIENTS OR LESS

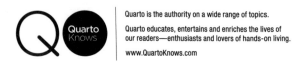

© 2015 Quarto Publishing Group USA Inc.

First published in the USA in 2015 by
Fair Winds Press, an imprint of
Quarto Publishing Group USA Inc.
100 Cummings Center, Suite 406-L
Beverly, MA 01915-6101
QuartoKnows.com
Visit our blogs at QuartoKnows.com.

19 18 17 16 15   1 2 3 4 5

ISBN: 978-1-59233-695-1

Digital edition published in 2015
eISBN: 978-1-62788-757-1

Library of Congress Cataloging-in-Publication
data available.

Cover and book design by
Laura H. Couallier, Laura Herrmann Design

Printed and bound in the United States.

*The information in this book is for educational purposes
only. It is not intended to replace the advice of a physician
or medical practitioner. Please see your health care
provider before beginning any new health program.*

Dedication

For my dear friends and next door neighbors, Keith Johnson and Peter Bane, who are passionate teachers of sustainable agriculture. For Joel Salatin of Polyface Farm, showing the world what agriculture can and should be, and for my friend Tom Tlusty and his partners at the Garden Tower Project, helping people grow their own organic food without having to own extensive acreage. For all who have fought for their right to raise poultry in their suburban neighborhoods or to grow vegetables instead of grass in their front yards. Indeed, to all who are changing the world and human health by teaching others how we can feed ourselves far better, without destroying the planet or giving our fate and our health over to multinational corporations.

Dana Carpender

PALEO/ PRIMAL

IN 5 INGREDIENTS OR LESS

More Than 200 Sugar-Free, Grain-Free, Gluten-Free Recipes

FAIR WINDS

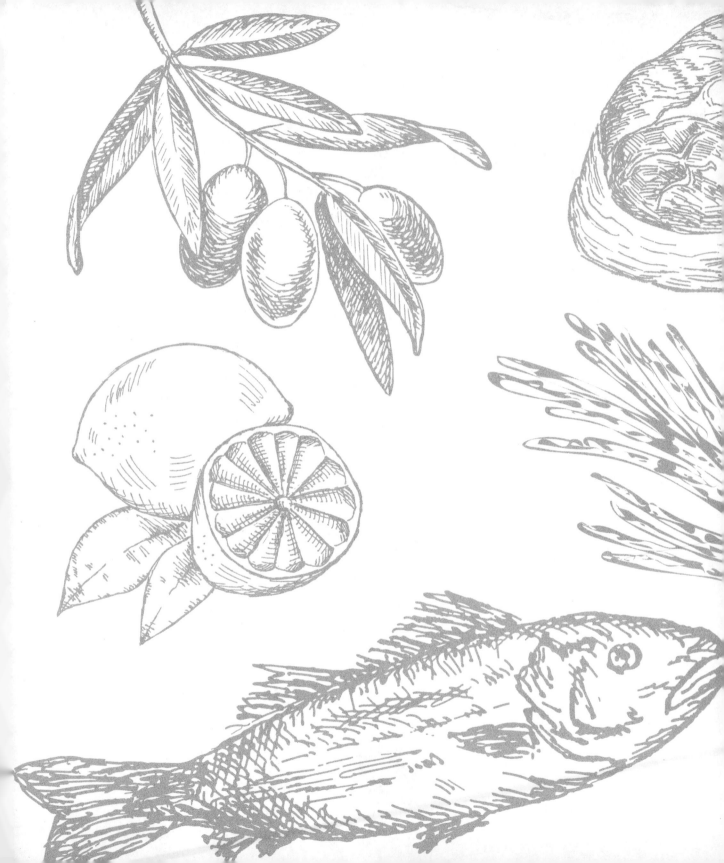

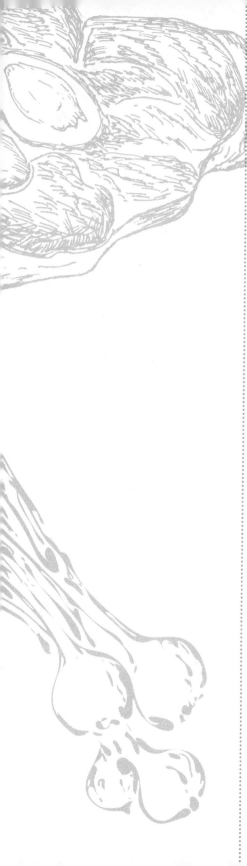

Contents

Paleo, Simplified

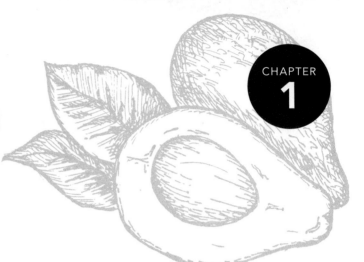

The concept of Paleo is so very simple. Paleo is the notion that we are healthiest eating those foods on which the human body evolved, the foods that our ancestors ate for an estimated two to three million years before the Agricultural Revolution roughly 10,000 years ago.

It is incredible to think that something like 75 percent of the "foods" in the average American grocery store didn't exist as recently as the Civil War.

Grains and beans have been around for a while, of course. Many people like to blame their deleterious effects on genetic modification.

In *Wheat Belly*, cardiologist William Davis, M.D., informed us of the alarming fact that, in wheat, simple hybridization—no gene splicing needed—results in novel genes, to the point where today's wheat is quite different, genetically, from that which our grandparents ate just a few decades ago.

Agriculture led humankind to quit following the herds and settle down, which led, in turn, to villages, specialization, and eventually civilization. It's hard to imagine how human history would have gone without it.

Agriculture was never, however, an unmixed blessing. Neolithic farmers were considerably shorter and weaker-boned than their hunter-gatherer forebears. Their teeth suffered, too, as they do to this day. Worse, women's pelvic outlets became smaller, making child-bearing both more painful and more dangerous. We have paid for architecture, art, and organization with our very bodies. It is interesting to contemplate how much of the history of medicine is a search for work-arounds for the problems caused by a sub-optimal diet.

It makes sense, then, that a move back in the direction of the diet that made our hunter-gatherer ancestors tall and strong would regain us some of that lost vitality.

Here is my assumption about you, dear reader: You've figured out that you feel a whole lot better when you eschew grains, especially gluten grains, sugar, corn syrup, and cheap vegetable oils. You've started eating clean—skipping chemical additives and buying organic when possible—adding more animal products, using traditional fats, and buying fresh, local, organic vegetables as much as possible. The farmers' market is your new social scene.

One problem: The rest of your life is the same as it ever was. You probably have the same job, kids, chauffeuring duties, and chores. Because all of those things remain the same, I bet you also still have the same need to occasionally do a little exercise and the same need to get sufficient sleep. (Indeed, one of the least-Paleo things we do in the modern world is regularly staying up long after dark. Get some sleep.)

Your Paleo ancestors very likely devoted a large chunk of their time to hunting, gathering, and preparing food. Certainly as recently as 150 years ago, food preparation was nearly a full-time task for at least one, and often more than one, person per household. Yet very few families now have a member who can devote every day to food prep.

Also, there's a good chance you're not an enthusiastic or experienced cook. I have known from the beginning of my career that, unlike many cookbook authors, my audience is not made up largely of "foodies," but rather of people who, until they realized the connection between what they were eating and their ill-health, had been living on macaroni and cheese dinners, carry-out pizza, cold cereal, and fast food like the rest of America.

In this chapter, I'll address common questions about the Paleo diet.

Which Foods Are Paleo or Primal?

These, to me, are the core principles of a Paleo diet.

- No grains, beans, or potatoes, nor anything that must be cooked to be edible, especially no gluten and no soy
- No refined or separated sugars
- No polyunsaturated vegetable oils

These, which Kurt Harris of the *Archevore* blog calls "Neolithic agents of disease" are the don'ts. I like to add this one "do":

- Eat plenty of animal protein and animal fats. There is no such thing as a vegetarian Paleo diet.

It has been interesting to watch the spread of the Paleo movement. People have different ideas about what "Paleo" means, about which foods are and which are not Paleo. It is confusing for me professionally. With no clear definition, some of you will find I've used ingredients you consider insufficiently "Paleo," while others will find that I have eschewed ingredients that you find acceptable. Heck, some of you will find I've done both. All I can do is explain my reasoning regarding what counts as Paleo and what does not: what I find most important and what I find less so.

Let's be clear on one thing: Virtually no one is eating a truly Paleolithic diet. Unless you're hunting and gathering local wild foods in season, you are eating differently than your Paleolithic ancestors did. There is nothing genuinely Paleo about eating coconut or lobster or avocados in the American Midwest, or lettuce in the winter, or drinking coffee most anywhere in the United States except possibly Hawaii.

Further, if you are in the United States, a gloriously interbred society, it's unlikely that you are living in the same sort of biosphere that your Paleolithic ancestors did, wherever they may have come from. Many of you have roots in widely spread places, and we know that hunter-gatherer diets varied considerably from place to place and from season to season. I could go out my back door and—were I skilled enough—hunt white-tailed deer, squirrel, opossum, raccoon, and wild turkey. I could gather hickory nuts, acorns, burdock root, persimmons, fox grapes, choke cherries, and ground cherries. This would be a pretty Paleo menu, but not for my English and Dutch ancestors, and certainly not for their deepest ancestors, who came—as did we all—from Africa, as the work of Paleoanthropologists Mary and Louis Leakey and their colleagues, and the discovery of Lucy, the oldest known human ancestor, in Ethiopia, have made plain.

Most of us are, of course, hunting for our foods at the grocery store, the health food store, and, if we're fortunate, the farmers' market. Even if you can afford to buy all organic, locally grown produce, it will have been bred for centuries for less bitterness, greater sweetness and juiciness, and larger fruits. If you buy all grass-fed or pasture-raised meat and eggs, they still will be from domesticated species.

They will also represent a far narrower spectrum of foods than our deep ancestors ate. Most grocery stores carry roughly a dozen kinds of meat and poultry, perhaps another dozen or so varieties of fish, and only one kind of egg. Most carry very few organ meats. Our ancestors ate pretty much anything that didn't eat them first, including insects, grubs, and eggs of every variety. Many cultures still do. These things, however, are hard to come by in my local grocery stores, and I suspect in yours as well.

I point this out not to suggest it is futile, but only to assert that the semi-religious fervor with which some people approach the Paleo lifestyle is misplaced. It is a heuristic, a tool, a way of looking at food and making choices. But it does little good to make it a series of complex laws that must be observed rigidly.

Here are my criteria for judging whether a food is "Paleo" or not, with some elaboration.

1. Is It Edible in Its Raw, Unprocessed Form?

Steak tartare, carpaccio, eggnog, and oysters on the half shell make it obvious that most animal foods are edible raw. This doesn't mean we *must* eat them raw, and it certainly doesn't eliminate the risk of bacteria or parasites in raw foods. (Our ancestors very probably had worms.) But it does mean that these are things our Paleolithic ancestors would have recognized as food.

Similarly, many roots and tubers, leaves and flowers, fruits, and nuts are edible just as they come from the earth, plant or tree, though you might want to wipe the dirt off first.

Grains and legumes, on the other hand, must be cooked to be edible. So must potatoes. You can eat a slice or two of raw potato without trouble, but if you eat a whole potato or two raw, you'll have a whale of a bellyache. It may even make you feel weak. (Greenish potatoes have "sun scald," and they are even higher in toxins, conceivably enough to be lethal.)

Toxins lurk elsewhere. Cashews come off the tree containing urushiol, the same toxin as poison ivy. The "raw" cashews you find at the health food store have actually been steamed to break this down. Tapioca, which I have seen used in some Paleo recipes, comes from the manioc or cassava root, which must be processed to remove toxins, including cyanide. If improperly processed, it can cause ataxia or paralysis. "Arrowroot," a starch many Paleo folks use in place of flour or cornstarch, actually comes from a variety of plants, one of which is the cassava. For this reason, and because it is a nutritionally void concentrated carbohydrate—virtually nothing but starch—I haven't used it. Canola oil comes from a hybridized version of a plant with the unfortunate name "rape." Rapeseed oil is toxic; historically it was used to make varnish. I can't consider these "we've-managed-to-make-it-nontoxic" things Paleo.

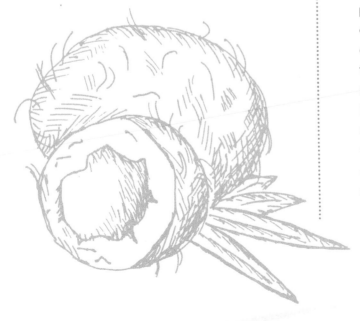

2. What Has Been Added to It?

I think we can all agree that Paleo foods should not resemble a chemistry experiment. We'll be avoiding artificial colors, flavors, sweeteners, preservatives, corn syrup, hydrogenated oils, and so on.

3. Has It Been Refined, Processed, or Both?

This is a somewhat fuzzy line. For example, I don't consider fruit juice Paleo, beyond a squeeze of citrus juice for flavoring, because the fiber has been removed—a refining process—allowing the consumption of dangerous quantities of sugar. However, I'm fine with coconut oil, from which the fiber has also been removed, and, for that matter, coconut flour, which is made from the fiber removed from the coconut oil. I'm also fine with stevia extracts. Call me inconsistent.

For that matter, all pure fats have been processed in some way, if only being pressed or rendered out of their sources. I avoid especially any fat that comes from a source that simply does not seem fatty. If I can't readily envision how the fat was extracted, I know it has to be processed to the point of damage. Further, I know that form of fat was never available in large quantities to our ancestors. These non-Paleo oils include soy, safflower, corn, and cottonseed.

In this book, I have also used some canned, bottled, and frozen foods. How do I rationalize this in the context of Paleo? Frozen is the easiest to explain. It's hard to imagine that Ice Age hunters didn't figure out that if they left the mammoth carcass out on the ice, preferably with a guard against scavengers, it would stay fresh a lot longer than it would in the cave, tent, or hut, where temperatures would run above freezing. Many frozen foods have all sorts of gunk added, but I don't see plain frozen vegetables as objectionable, or, for that matter, the meat in my sizeable freezer.

But what about canning, jarring, and bottling? These are unquestionably post-Paleolithic technologies. On the other hand, as Grandma could have told you, they allow the preservation of food with no additives. Just because many, if not most, canned or bottled foods are a Festival of Garbage doesn't mean they have to be.

The benefit of admitting carefully selected canned, jarred, or bottled foods in the context of limiting the number of ingredients in a recipe is obvious. Using organic jarred salsa lets us add tomatoes, onions, garlic, cumin, and other seasonings to a dish with only one ingredient. Likewise, organic, additive-free, pasta, pizza, and hot sauces give us tremendous flavoring bang for our ingredient buck. Happily, these are proliferating in number and becoming far easier to find. I will give you the names of the specific brands I use for these recipes, but do yourself a favor and spend 15 minutes reading labels every now and then, especially at the health food store. You will uncover products that will let you add complex flavors without adding objectionable ingredients.

One form of processing and refining that people seldom consider is the consumption of only muscle meats. I get snarky about weight loss articles that recommend "whole foods" such as boneless, skinless chicken breast. I have thirty-odd chickens in my backyard, and every one of them has bones and skin, not to mention organs. It will behoove you nutritionally to make an effort to eat more of the animal—such as some of the tougher cuts of meat, organ meats and skin, and some marrow and to make bones into broth. (I eat a lot of chicken wings, which offer lots of skin, gelatin, and fat along with the meat and lovely bones for broth. You know the pointy little bit at the end that gets thrown away? I actually roast those quite crisp and chew 'em up, bone and all.)

What About Dairy?

This, dear reader, is where "Paleo" becomes "primal." As popularized by superstar blogger and World's Hottest Sixty-Something Guy, Mark Sisson (I've met Mark, and yeah, he really does look that good), "primal" basically comes down to Paleo-plus-quality-dairy. It's an idea that has caught on with many people in the ancestral nutrition movement. (If you've somehow missed Mark's stuff, it's at marksdailyapple.com.)

I would argue that mankind has been eating cheese since we became hunters, which was the step that some scientists believe was instrumental in our becoming truly human. (If you're as geeky as I am, look up the Expensive Tissue Hypothesis. It's fascinating stuff.) When you kill a baby ruminant—a goat, sheep, buffalo, or whatever—you will find cheese curds in its stomach. Did our ancestors throw these away? I very much doubt it. My guess is that the jump from following the herds as hunters, to keeping herds for both meat and dairy, came when some cheese-curd-eating genius thought, "Wait. We could get food from the same goat over and over!"

Whether you tolerate dairy well or not will largely be a matter of genealogy. The further back your ancestors started dairying, the more likely you are to tolerate dairy well. My ancestors are mostly English, with a little Dutch thrown in, cheese-eaters all. I have no trouble with dairy.

Many people who skip cheese and yogurt eat grass-fed butter or ghee—clarified butter—with no trouble. Because butter and ghee are terrific sources of vitamins, antioxidants, and astoundingly healthful fats, including conjugated linoleic acid (CLA), noted in the *American Journal of Clinical Nutrition* in 2004 as potentially controlling body fat deposition, reducing inflammation, and strengthening immunity, I consider this a fine idea.

The availability of high-quality dairy will depend on where you live. Here in Southern Indiana, there are many small farms. I can get local grass-fed cheese, both from cow's milk and goat's milk, some raw, some not. I can get local grass-fed butter, as well. Raw milk is illegal here, but there is a dairy that produces unhomogenized milk, which means the cream rises to the top, that is minimally pasteurized, in other words, heated to the minimum legal temperature for the shortest legal length of time. Check your local health food stores to see what's available.

More and more big chains are carrying the Kerrygold brand of Irish grass-fed dairy products. I buy their butter and cheese at local grocery stores and in larger packages at Costco. (Go to http://kerrygoldusa.com/find_us/ to find a source near you.)

In this book, I have included dairy when I felt it really "made" the recipe. In some cases, I have given alternatives for those of you who are dairy-free. But the vast majority of these recipes do not include dairy.

How Can I Find Balance?

When eating differently from the people around us, it is helpful to give some thought to priorities. We all have moments when we are not completely in control of our food, whether it is at a truck stop or Mom's house. For many of us, too, cost is an issue. Knowing your own priorities will help you decide between better and worse when perfect is not an option.

My most important priority is keeping my carb load quite low. I have tried adding limited Paleo carbs, such as sweet potatoes, back to my diet, and I have been rewarded with weight gain and a noticeable deterioration in my bloodwork. Indeed, as I put the finishing touches on this book, I'm about a half size bigger than when I started, simply from Paleo carbs. Carbohydrate tolerance varies widely, however. If you have no blood sugar issues, have never been obese, and/or are a natural athlete, this may not be a priority for you.

My second priority is keeping gluten out of my diet. I have no reason to believe I am especially gluten sensitive, but I am convinced that the stuff is not wholesome. Indeed, I am convinced that it is dangerous. I avoid all grains, and I consider gluten-bearing grains to be especially harmful.

Close behind is my third priority of avoiding trans fats and objectionable oils, including safflower, soy, canola, and cottonseed and other highly processed, omega-6-rich seed oils.

For me, those are the Big Three. Beyond that, I do what I can, you know? Here are a few other guidelines I follow in my own life.

Because I live outside of town and have a huge yard, I have thirty-odd chickens supplying me with excellent eggs. When egg production slows down in the winter, I spend the extra money for local small farm eggs rather than buying grocery store eggs.

I buy grass-fed local meat and dairy and Kerrygold butter and cheeses as much as I can afford, but I will eat conventionally raised animal products.

Some of my produce comes from the local farmers' market and some from Keith and Peter, my Organic Gardening God next door neighbors. Their yard is a wonder to behold. But I buy produce from the grocery store, too, keeping the "Dirty Dozen Plus" and "Clean Fifteen" from the Environmental Working Group (EWG) in mind. The EWG has compounded lists of the varieties of produce most and least likely to be contaminated with pesticides and other noxious chemicals. These were originally called the "Dirty Dozen" and the "Clean Fifteen," but both lists have since been expanded. If your food budget is tight, it makes sense to buy organic when purchasing items from the first list and to save money by purchasing conventionally grown produce when buying foods on the second list.

Try to Buy These Foods Organic

First, let's talk about the foods to watch out for. These are the foods that are most likely to be heavily contaminated, ranked in order, from dirtiest to least objectionable. If you're trying to leverage your organic food dollar, these are the items where it will most serve you to pony up the bucks.

1. Peaches
2. Apples
3. Sweet bell peppers
4. Celery
5. Nectarines
6. Strawberries
7. Cherries
8. Pears
9. Grapes (imported)
10. Spinach
11. Lettuce
12. Potatoes
13. Carrots
14. Green beans
15. Hot peppers
16. Cucumbers
17. Raspberries
18. Plums
19. Grapes (domestic)
20. Oranges

OK to Buy Conventional

I am happy to report that the list of fruits and vegetables least likely to be badly contaminated has expanded to twenty one items. According to the EWG, the following produce has the lowest pesticide load, ranked in order with the produce with the absolute lowest pesticides first.

1. Onion
2. Avocado
3. Sweet corn (frozen)
4. Pineapples
5. Mango
6. Asparagus
7. Sweet peas (frozen)
8. Kiwi
9. Bananas
10. Cabbage
11. Broccoli
12. Papaya
13. Blueberries
14. Cauliflower
15. Winter squash
16. Watermelon
17. Sweet potatoes
18. Tomatoes
19. Honeydew melon
20. Canteloupe
21. Mushrooms

Because of these lists, I buy organic berries, lettuce, celery, and apples, but I will buy the cheap onions in the net sack, conventional cabbage (always dirt cheap), and the big, pretty heads of cauliflower. I buy avocados at Aldi, my cheapest local source.

Your priority list may be different, but it will save you stress if you give it some thought in advance. It will help with decision making when faced with a mother determined to feed you all your childhood favorites or the snack selection at a gas station mini-mart.

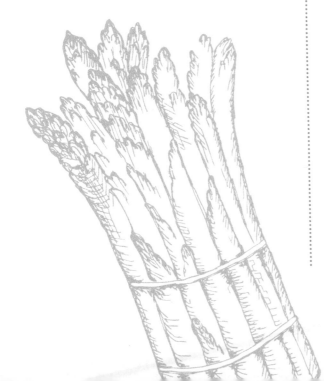

What About Sweeteners?

Regular use of sweeteners in pretty much any form cannot be considered truly Paleo, or even primal, despite the proliferation of Paleo/primal dessert recipes. However, having grown up, as we all have, with sweetened foods forming a pathological percentage of our diet, it is unlikely we're going to simply quit eating them all together. So let's take a look at the contenders.

Agave Nectar

I put this first because if you read nothing else in this section, I want you to get this message loud and clear: *Agave nectar is not Paleo. It is not natural. It is not healthful.* Agave nectar is the most egregious fraud perpetrated upon the nutrition-conscious community since I became interested in nutrition in 1978.

The word "nectar" summons up idyllic images of simply tapping the plant. Hah. Instead, agave nectar is produced remarkably like high fructose corn syrup: The longer chain carbohydrates in the agave plant, in this case fructooligosaccharides, a sweet fiber, are broken down into their component sugars using enzymes, in a factory. (For corn syrup, the same sort of enzyme digestion process is used on cornstarch.) The resulting syrup is higher in fructose than high fructose corn syrup; and therefore, it is even worse for you.

You know why agave nectar has a low glycemic index? Because fructose has to be processed by the liver before it is absorbed, subjecting it to a metabolic bottleneck. This means that fructose is very hard on your liver. Indeed, in their book *The 6-Week Cure for the Middle-Aged Middle*, Michael Eades, M.D., and Mary Dan Eades, M.D., assert that fructose is the biggest cause of non-alcoholic fatty liver disease (NAFLD). Frighteningly, Harvard Medical School says NAFLD was "virtually unknown before 1980," but now it affects as much as 30 percent of the population and a whopping 70 to 90 percent of the obese and diabetic. They blame the dramatic increase in fructose consumption in the past several decades. The Gout and Uric Acid Education Society recommends limiting fructose.

In 2010, Anthony Heaney, M.D., Ph.D., of UCLA's Jonsson Comprehensive Cancer Center, having studied the differing effects of glucose and fructose on pancreatic cancer cells and finding that the cells used the fructose to generate the nucleic acids needed to proliferate, stated "…these findings show that cancer cells can readily metabolize fructose to increase proliferation. They have major significance for cancer patients, given dietary refined fructose." The American Heart Association singles out fructose in elevating triglycerides, saying, "Foods that contain high amounts of simple sugars, especially fructose, raise triglyceride levels." And a 2014 article in *The Journal of Nutritional Biochemistry* states that "Fructose overconsumption has been involved in the genesis and progression of the metabolic syndrome," concluding "We propose that high-fructose-diet-induced alterations of glucocorticoid signaling in both hypothalamus and adipose tissue result in enhanced adipogenesis …" In other words, fructose makes you fat. Skip the agave nectar.

Honey

Raw, unfiltered honey is undeniably natural, and it was likely the only concentrated sweet some of our hunter-gatherer ancestors ever ate. But how often did they eat it? How often did hunter-gatherers find a bee tree? Having found one, what did they do? Keep in mind that they didn't have jars, and they were, in most cases, nomadic. How could they have stored and carried something as fluid, sticky, and heavy as honey?

I suspect that discovering a bee tree was an occasion for a party, where everyone gorged themselves on the sugary treat and put on a few pounds. But to take honey along and use it in everyday cooking, assuming they were even cooking? Put it in beverages? Bake it into cookies and cakes? I see little Paleo about that.

It is also well to remember that even raw, unfiltered honey is virtually entirely sugar, with the same breakdown as table sugar. Both are a 50/50 blend of glucose and fructose. Honey will spike blood sugar and trigger insulin surges just as effectively as table sugar.

None of this is to say you mustn't eat honey. If you were born with a robust carbohydrate metabolism, honey will be one of your sweeteners of choice. Just don't fool yourself into thinking that going through a jar a week is fine because "It's Paleo!"

Maple Syrup

This one is iffier. Forty gallons (151 L) of maple sap boil down to just 1 gallon (3.8 L) of maple syrup. Surely that calls for as much technology as cooking grains and beans. Still, you can drink maple sap raw, and again, maple syrup has a reputation for being "natural," so some Paleo folks use it. I've included maple syrup in a few recipes, largely for its incomparable flavor. Like honey, maple syrup has a few nutrients in it, but it derives 99 percent of its calories from sugar. Govern yourself accordingly.

If you'd like to avoid the sugar in maple syrup, you can use sugar-free pancake syrup. It's definitely not Paleo, but it works well. Or you can use a combination of erythritol and natural maple extract. The one I have is Boyajian pure maple extract. I bought it on Amazon.com, and it's excellent.

Sucanat

This is unrefined sugar cane juice that has been dried and ground to a coarse powder. It tastes a lot like brown sugar, although the texture is different. I don't think it's strictly Paleo, but it seems as Paleo as maple syrup to me. Folks who live where sugar cane is grown have long chewed on the cane itself as a sweet treat. I've offered sucanat as an alternative in just a couple of recipes. Health food stores should carry it.

Erythritol

What the heck is this, and how can I consider it Paleo? Erythritol is one of the sugar alcohol or polyol class of sweeteners. It's a carbohydrate, but one that is neither digested nor absorbed. Therefore, it has no effect on blood sugar and can be discounted by carb counters. (This is not true of all the sugar alcohols. About half of maltitol, sorbitol, and xylitol is absorbed.) Unlike other sugar alcohols, erythritol has virtually no gastric effect, so there's no gas and no laxative effect.

Erythritol occurs naturally in some fruits and fermented foods, so it's not a total newcomer to the human diet, although like all concentrated sweeteners, the quantity is greater than our ancestors would have eaten. Commercially, erythritol is created by fermentation of glucose.

When I worked on a sugar-free, grain-free cookbook, *CarbSmart Grain-Free, Sugar-Free Living Cookbook,* with Caitlin Weeks, a.k.a. *Grass-Fed Girl,* I noticed she used birch xylitol in her recipes, which has about as much claim to being Paleo as erythritol because most people probably didn't chew on birch logs. Because xylitol is partially absorbed, it does have a gastric effect, so I consider it a less desirable choice (though it also apparently improves dental health). I asked Caitlin why xylitol instead of erythritol and why specifically birch xylitol. She replied that she could be sure that birch xylitol had no GMOs.

Well, that was easily dealt with. A quick search on Amazon.com turned up erythritol with no GMOs, so I bought a bag. At this writing, it's running $37 for 5 pounds (2.3 kg), and I haven't used even half of that working on this book.

Erythritol has the interesting property of being endothermic. It absorbs energy when wet, creating a cooling effect. This works better in some applications than others. I often combine erythritol with stevia to get the sweetness I want while minimizing the cooling effect. You can buy commercially available sweeteners that combine erythritol and stevia, Truvia being the best known. I'm just not crazy about the stuff.

By the way, if you'd like a powdered sugar substitute, you can run granular erythritol through your food processor for a few minutes.

Stevia

Stevia is a South American shrub with very sweet leaves. That sweetness comes not from sugar, but from *steviosides*, naturally occurring super-sweet compounds exclusive to the stevia plant. This means that stevia is virtually carb-free, with no effect on blood sugar.

Unlike honey, the stevia shrub isn't guarded by bees, and unlike maple syrup, it doesn't require fire, huge vats, and long, tedious boiling to yield a useful sweetener.

You can buy dried stevia leaves, and this would be the most authentically Paleo form. The leaves are also hard to use, with a flavor some compare to licorice and a bitter aftertaste. I mostly use them for sweetening herbal teas.

The form of stevia I find easiest to use and consider acceptably Paleo is liquid stevia extract. This comes in dropper bottles. It is generally blended either with water, glycerin (a fraction of fat, so hardly a stranger to the human diet), or alcohol. The alcohol extracts have so little alcohol per drop that it should have virtually no impact on your body. Liquid stevia comes both plain and in flavors. I use flavored liquid stevia all of the time; it is a staple in my kitchen. My plain liquid stevia is from NuNaturals, while the flavored stuff is either NOW "Better Stevia" brand or SweetLeaf brand, but I see no reason why other brands shouldn't work fine. I buy mine at local health food stores. You can also buy liquid stevia online.

It's important to know the sweetness equivalency of your stevia. The brands I use run about:

6 drops = 1 teaspoon sugar in sweetness

I generally substitute the following:

¼ teaspoon of liquid stevia for ¼ cup (50 g) sugar
½ teaspoon liquid stevia for ½ cup (100 g) sugar, etc.

In many recipes, I have combined honey with liquid stevia. The honey adds texture, and the stevia brings the recipe up to the desired sweetness without additional sugar. I have also combined stevia with erythritol to reduce the cooling effect of the erythritol.

Yacon Syrup

Yacon syrup, similar to molasses, is derived from a South American root. Because about half of it consists of fructooligosaccharides, a sweet prebiotic fiber, it is easier on blood sugar than many syrups. It is just starting to show up in health food stores, but is available online.

Monk Fruit

Also called *lo han guo,* monk fruit is a Chinese fruit. Its extract is 300 times sweeter than sugar. Traditional Chinese Medicine uses monk fruit to treat obesity and diabetes. I haven't used monk fruit in these recipes, but in any of them where I have used plain stevia extract, you can use monk fruit extract instead. NuNaturals makes a monk fruit extract, which contains only *lo han guo,* water, and glycerin. EZ Sweetz makes a stevia-monk fruit blend that I like as well, although it contains some sodium benzoate and potassium sorbate. The quantity in a few drops strikes me as negligible. As always, you'll want to know the sweetness equivalence to sugar. The EZ Sweetz is considerably sweeter than the NuNaturals.

Fruit

Fruit can lend sweetness to dishes, and I've used various fruits for that purpose in this book. Again, the sweetness in fruit comes from sugar, although fruit is not the concentrated source of sugar that honey or maple syrup are. If you've got blood sugar trouble, you'll want to keep an eye on even this source of sugar.

Decide for yourself which is more important, Paleo authenticity or keeping your blood sugar down, and make your choices accordingly. If you have blood sugar problems, your glucometer is your friend. Let it guide you.

What About Salt?

Some Paleo peeps shun salt altogether. But despite demonization, salt is an essential nutrient. A serious salt deficiency will kill you. The question is, would our hunter-gatherer ancestors have had access to salt?

Surely they would have been aware of mineral-rich areas. Places where the soil is salty, known as "salt licks," draw game from far around, and they would have been prime hunting grounds. Seeing animals licking the ground, Ogg would have tasted the soil. I find it likely that salt deposits would have been discovered this way.

Anyone who lived near salt water would have known that the white stuff left behind by drying tide pools had the coveted flavor. For that matter, people who lived by bodies of salt water would have gotten plenty of salt eating raw clams, mussels, oysters, and other shellfish.

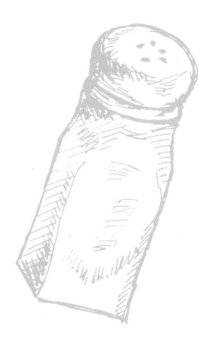

I suspect that anywhere that salt could be found, our ancestors found it and ate it. We know that salt was one of the earliest trade commodities. Is it hard to believe that nomads whose travels brought them near a salt cave or salt water would take salt along, both for their own use and to trade with other tribes?

By avoiding processed, packaged foods, you will automatically remove most of the salt from your diet.

That brings me to the topic of balance. The sodium in your diet needs to be balanced with potassium. If your intake of vegetables, fruits, pork, and fish, which are all rich in potassium, increases, you will need enough sodium to balance it.

Diets high in carbohydrates stimulate insulin release. The journal *Nutrition and Metabolism* refers to carbohydrate as "the major secretagogue of insulin"—thus causing the body to retain sodium. As long ago as 1992, an article titled "Effects of Insulin on Renal Sodium Excretion" in the journal *Hypertension* stated that "the ability of insulin to decrease urinary sodium excretion has been recognized for more than 30 years." Carbohydrate restriction lowers insulin levels, allowing the body to eliminate sodium properly.

In *The Art and Science of Low Carbohydrate Living*, researchers Stephen Phinney, M.D., Ph.D., and Jeff Volek, Ph.D., R.D., state that people who cut out concentrated carbohydrates—starches and sugars—often find themselves weak and tired, not from lack of carbs, but from lack of sodium.

However, grocery store salt is refined to eliminate all minerals except for sodium and chlorine, often with iodine added as well. (The iodine is beneficial; it's the other additives and the lack of trace minerals I object to.) Sea salt, on the other hand, contains a wide variety of trace minerals. There's just one problem: Our seas and oceans are sadly polluted. There is, however, a way around this: mined sea salt. All around the world, there are deposits of salt that are remnants of ancient seas. This salt was deposited long before mankind was around, much less had a chance to dump chemicals in the oceans. This is the finest, most nutritious, and most Paleo salt you can use.

I use a brand called Real Salt that's mined in Utah, while friends of mine favor salt from deposits in the Himalayas. (How long ago did an ocean have to dry up to have left salt in the Himalayas?) Any salt from ancient deposits should be fine, so long as nothing is added. Your ancient sea bed salt will not be pure white. The salt I buy is pale pink, as is a lot of Himalayan salt. Pure white salt is suspect.

Because you're not using iodized salt, make sure you're getting iodine elsewhere. If you eat a lot of seafood—fresh water fish doesn't count—that may be enough. Seaweed is also an excellent source of iodine, if you're fond of it. I take a few drops of Lugol's solution, which is a combination of iodine and potassium iodide, in my tea every morning.

Can I Have Alcohol and Vinegar?

Some Paleo folks allow for alcohol and vinegar, but others do not. I have used them here, although I have avoided grain-derived alcohol and vinegars.

Wild yeasts are everywhere; carbohydrates ferment. Park rangers tell stories of bears finding fruit that has fermented on the bush or vine and eating enough to get drunk. If bears did it, so did Ogg. He didn't have bottles of the stuff around the cave, but they are not foreign substances that are toxic unless cooked. (Alcohol is toxic if you drink enough of it, but ½ cup (120 ml) of wine in a dish to be shared by four people does not strike me as dangerous.)

Vinegar is the natural end product of alcohol, unless it is distilled first. At my old house, we had an apple tree in the backyard; some of the apples that fell to the ground smelled of vinegar. Do you think a hungry caveman would have passed them up? I don't.

Do You Use Flour Substitutes?

Almond meal and coconut flour are the flour substitutes I have used. Both are widely available in health food stores and often in regular grocery stores as well. The widely-distributed Bob's Red Mill brand includes both.

I often make my own almond meal, simply by running shelled almonds through my food processor until it reaches cornmeal texture. This can be subbed for the commercial version, but it takes a decent food processor. (If you don't have a really good food processor, consider buying one. I've had a $30 Black and Decker and a $125 Cuisinart, and there's no question which is the better, more powerful, more versatile machine.)

Coconut flour is milled from coconut that has first been pressed for its oil. Putting shredded coconut through your food processor will not give you coconut flour. (It will, however, give you coconut butter, a.k.a. coconut manna.) You have to purchase it.

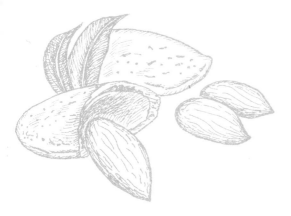

Which Fats Are Paleo?

Fat has been reviled for so long that it can take a while to wrap our heads around the idea that proper, traditional fats are one of the most valuable foods we can eat. Most of the vegetable oils we've been told are "healthy" are anything but. I have used only the following few, carefully chosen fats in this book.

Lard

For a long time, lard was the most widely used cooking fat in the United States. Only in the twentieth century did the marketing of vegetable oils move lard out of its central position. It deserves a place in your kitchen.

We're talking proper lard, that is: unprocessed lard from pastured pigs. Even if you're eating grocery store meat, seek out a source of proper lard. Don't even consider buying the stuff in the grocery store. The grocery store junk has a less favorable fatty acid balance, and it's been bleached. It's also usually hydrogenated, the process that creates trans fats.

Proper lard, on the other hand, is a lovely blend of monounsaturated and saturated fats. It's as healthful as can be. It's also one of the best dietary sources of vitamin D. Turns out, pigs make vitamin D in their skin on sun exposure, just like we do, and that vitamin D is stored in the fat.

I buy lard in 5-pound (2.3 kg) buckets from a local small farm. At this writing, I pay $14, or just under $3 per pound (455 g). It's absolutely worth it. Any time I want a bland fat—for sautéing, pan-broiling, basting, or what-have-you—I reach for my lard. I keep the main bucket in my deep freeze to keep it fresh. I scoop out enough for about a week at a time into a smaller jar that I keep by the stove.

Bacon Grease

If you've spent the money for nitrate-free bacon from pasture-raised pigs, do not, for the love of all that's holy, throw away the grease. That's manna from heaven, as delicious as it is good for you. It has a similar fatty acid profile to lard, of course. I confess to saving the grease from grocery store bacon, as well. My bacon grease lives in an old salsa jar by the stove. I use it up before it goes bad. I use it to fry eggs, sauté vegetables, baste things—all sorts of fatty uses.

Coconut Oil

Coconut oil is one of the most saturated fats available. Despite propaganda, that's a good thing. Why? Because saturated fats are extremely stable. Unlike polyunsaturated fats, they don't go rancid easily. Coconut oil will keep for a year without refrigeration, even when open. Saturated fats do not cause inflammation in the body. Interestingly, they also help remove fat from your liver, according to Michael and Mary Dan Eades, the doctors who wrote *Protein Power*.

Coconut oil has other benefits. It's loaded with lauric acid, a fatty acid that kills yeasts and fungi. Indeed, coconut oil has long been used by nutritionists and some doctors to treat systemic candida infection. Research conducted by the Department of Medical Microbiology and Parasitology at the University College Hospital, Ibadan, Nigeria, and published in the *Journal of Medicinal Food* backs this up. Coconut oil stimulates the thyroid, which can help with weight loss. It also has a very high content of medium-chain triglycerides (MCT). These fats can be used directly as fuel by the muscles and so can be used for quick energy, without the let-down sugar brings. Studies done in Japan and reported in *The Journal of Nutritional Science and Vitaminology* showed that athletes given MCT showed an increase both in intensity and duration of exercise.

You can buy two kinds of coconut oil: extra virgin coconut oil and just plain coconut oil. The extra virgin is simply pressed from coconut meat with no processing. It is extremely healthful, but it also has a distinct coconut aroma, which may or may not work with the recipe you're planning. There is also just plain coconut oil, which is widely used in Indian cuisine. It's more processed, but it still resists rancidity, will clear fat out of your liver, and provide quick energy to your muscles. It's also quite bland, which makes it suitable for a wider range of cooking purposes. It's up to you how strict you want to be. I think both are useful to keep on hand.

Palm Oil

Palm oil is popular with many Paleo folks. Like coconut oil, it is highly saturated and therefore quite stable. Nutritionally, it is acceptable. However, palm oil agriculture is resulting in the slaughter of orangutans. I cannot use it in good conscience.

MCT Oil

Some Paleo folks use MCT (medium chain triglyceride) oil, a liquid oil derived from coconut oil. It has the advantage of being both bland and liquid at room temperature. And, as mentioned earlier, it can be used directly for fuel by the muscles. If you decide to buy MCT oil, shop around. I've seen widely varying prices. I mostly order mine from Puritan's Pride, a large mail order supplement house.

MCT oil is not strictly Paleo, but it appears to be more healthful than most of the bland liquid oils. Substitute light olive oil or high-heat organic sunflower oil if you like, but these are both refined to some degree as well. Or use extra-virgin olive oil and accept that your mayonnaise or whatever will be pretty olive-y.

Olive Oil

Olive oil is not authentically Paleo, but it has a very long history of use, and it appears to be pretty benign. The Paleo community has, for the very most part, embraced it. It is useful because most saturated fats are not liquid at room temperature, making them unsuitable for salad dressings and the like. If you're looking for a Mediterranean flavor, olive oil is essential.

I've used two grades of olive oil: extra-virgin olive oil and light olive oil. Extra virgin is more nutritious, but it does have a pronounced flavor. This is wonderful in many uses, but occasionally I want a blander liquid fat. In these cases, I use light olive oil. The fatty acid balance, which I consider essential, is not substantially affected by the refining process used to make light olive oil. However, it is up to you whether you wish to use this more refined oil and to decide if the stronger flavor of the extra-virgin olive oil will suit you in, say, mayonnaise.

Avocado Oil

Logically enough, this is oil pressed from avocados, and it's healthful stuff. It has a much less assertive flavor than olive oil, and so it is helpful when you want a liquid oil that won't take over a dish.

There are other Paleo fats. Indeed, the fat of any grass-fed or pastured meat is healthful and valuable for cooking. Tallow (beef dripping), chicken fat, and fat from roasted marrow are all worth keeping and using as cooking fat. I didn't use them in these recipes because, for the most part, they can't be purchased, but rather they have to be rendered in your kitchen. I'm guessing most of you don't want the hassle.

Milk Substitutes and Eggs

Here are notes about three popular ingredients.

Almond Milk

Some Paleo cookbooks call for almond milk, but all the packaged almond milk I have found is replete with additives. I don't see what is "Paleo" about something so processed. Accordingly, I have not used it here.

Coconut Milk

It is entirely possible to make coconut milk at home; I have done it. It's kind of a pain, but you can do it. However, I use canned coconut milk, generally Thai Kitchen brand or Kroger's store brand. Both of these have a gum thickener, which is not "Paleo kosher." A few brands of canned coconut milk contain nothing but coconut and water; if it matters to you, read the labels.

All of these recipes were developed using full-fat coconut milk. Coconut oil is very healthful stuff, and my body is happiest on a high-fat diet, so low-fat coconut milk simply makes no sense for me. You can try it if you prefer, but I can't vouch for the results.

Some coconut milk comes in 13.5-ounce (380 ml) cans, and others come in 14-ounce (410 ml) cans. A half ounce more or less is not going to make a difference in any of these recipes.

I have looked at the thinner coconut milks in cartons in the dairy section. I fail to see how these are more Paleo than locally raised, grass-fed cow's milk.

Eggs

A few recipes in this book call for raw eggs. This runs directly counter to the food safety information we've had drummed into our heads for the past couple of decades. According to the Centers for Disease Control and Prevention, only one out of every 20,000 uncracked, properly refrigerated eggs is actually contaminated. As one woman I talked with a long time ago with degrees in public health and food science put it, "The risk is less than the risk of breaking your leg on any given trip down the stairs." That's with factory farmed eggs. I consider small farm eggs —and the eggs from my backyard—even safer.

It's not that there's no risk in eating eggs; there's a risk to everything. But I'm increasingly convinced that people worry about the wrong things. They get panicky about eating raw eggs or raw milk while consuming Coca-Cola, Lucky Charms, and Wonder Bread. For what it's worth, I've never gotten sick from a raw egg.

If you're unhappy about raw eggs, you can pasteurize them. You'll need a digital thermometer. Put the eggs in a saucepan and cover them with water. Heat the water on high to 140°F (60°C). Hold the eggs at that temperature—and no hotter—for 3 minutes. Then immediately pour off the hot water and flush the eggs with several changes of cold water. Use the eggs right away or store them in the refrigerator until needed.

Can You Use Packaged Foods in Paleo Recipes?

I've been cooking since I had to stand on a step stool to reach the stove; it comes as naturally to me as breathing. I like to layer flavors, adding a little of this and a little of that. Grabbing that extra ingredient—or two, or three—is instinct. But I do not write recipes for me; I write them for *you*. I have long known that, unlike a lot of cookbook authors, my audience is not made up largely of hard-core foodies. Many of you don't have much time to cook. Many of you simply don't have the inclination.

This is where many cookbooks have you reaching for baking mix, canned biscuits, or flavored rice mix, to get full, layered flavors with a minimum of ingredients. I do not have that luxury, nor do I want it. I don't eat that stuff, and neither should you.

On the other hand, hard-core Paleo can be a rigorous road. Surely there must be something between "mix seasoned rice and noodle mix with canned cream of mushroom soup" and "you must make every single thing entirely from scratch, with fresh, locally sourced ingredients." We will walk this middle path in this book.

In service to the middle path, I have done a lot of label-reading, looking for products that serve our no-junk needs—that have no grain; sugar; cheap soy, canola, or safflower oil; trans fats; or artificial flavors—while allowing us to make family-pleasing dishes with a reasonable amount of effort. I deemed acceptable dried garlic and onion and spices, some spice "extractives," and citric acid, which is found in citrus fruits, of course. I chose products that lacked the "organic" label but had no added sugar, over products that were organic, but had "organic" sugar, cane juice, and the like.

You will, of course, decide for yourself where to draw the line. If you have a stronger carb metabolism than I, you may decide that a tiny quantity of organic sugar beats nonorganic tomatoes. The following are some products I used in developing these recipes. I recommend you do some label-reading yourself when you have a free hour or two. You may be surprised at what you find!

Salsa: This is, hands-down, the most useful packaged ingredient in this book, allowing you to add tomato, onion, garlic, and cumin all in one. This works for Mexican food and also for curry. Many salsas include sugar, so read the labels. I used both regular "chunky" salsa and chipotle salsa. I found more acceptable salsas in my local grocery stores than at health food stores because a lot of health food brands include organic sugar or evaporated cane juice. My local store brand salsas, Marsh's store brand chunky salsa, and President's Choice Chipotle Salsa at Kroger do not have added sugar. Go figure.

Some health food stores carry freshly made salsa; keep your eyes open. If you have a Trader Joe's near you, they have at least a couple of salsas that work for us.

Pasta sauce: Similar to salsa, pasta sauce lets us add a broad flavor palate with one ingredient. The things to look out for here are sugar, corn syrup, and objectionable oils. Too many "health food" brands include soy oil, which is seriously not Paleo. I used Kirkland Signature Marinara Sauce from Costco. I also found Rao's Homemade Arrabiata Sauce, a hot and spicy pasta sauce that adds a great zing. Both of these have no added sugar, and they use olive oil, not soy, safflower, or canola.

Pesto: In many recipes, a blend of basil, garlic, and Parmesan hits exactly the right note. Read labels to find pesto made with all olive oil. If you are dairy-free, you'll find a recipe for Anchovy-Walnut Pesto on page 34. It works in any recipe calling for pesto!

Harissa: My new culinary love is harissa, a North African condiment of hot peppers and spices. Often harissa contains junk, but I have discovered Mina brand, which is delicious and blessedly free of junk. It is not blow-the-top-of-your-head-off hot, just pleasantly spicy. Sahara Mart, my local international/gourmet/health food grocery, carries Mina Harissa, but if you can't find it locally, you can buy it online.

Spice blends: Before buying spice blends, check the labels for sugar, artificial flavors, and MSG, among other pitfalls. I found great seasoned salt, from the Real Salt company, at Bloomingfoods, the local health food coop, and a McCormick Gourmet Mediterranean Style Sea Salt Grinder at Costco. Both of these are available online too. I also made liberal use of good old Italian seasoning, simply a blend of herbs. Keep an eye out for spice blends with clean ingredients. Few things will let you vary your cookery more easily.

Hot sauce: Many hot sauces contain sugar, including some of the most popular. Happily, I found sugarless versions of Louisiana-style hot sauce, chipotle hot sauce, and sriracha sauce. Frank's Hot Sauce, widely available, is a Louisiana-style hot sauce similar to original Tabasco, but with no sugar. Melinda's Hot Sauces makes an excellent chipotle sauce. And at Bloomingfoods, our local food coop, I found Dark Star sriracha, to fill all your sriracha urges. If you can't find Melinda's Chipotle or Dark Star sriracha, once again, they're available online.

Guacamole: Wholly Guacamole brand is pretty clean and widely available. Best of all, it comes in 2-ounce (55 g) single-serving cups. Any good health food grocery should have an acceptable brand of guacamole available and some regular grocery stores will as well.

Canned or jarred tomatoes and tomato paste: I use canned or jarred diced tomatoes, tomato puree, and tomato paste in a few recipes. Look for organic products, in BPA-free cans, and even better, glass jars.

Canned fish: Various recipes in this book include canned anchovies, sardines, tuna, and clams. For the first three, I have used the versions canned in olive oil. Clams I found canned only with salt and clam juice. Look for 'em. Pay for 'em. It's worth it. Anchovies, in particular, are a wildly versatile seasoning. Used judiciously, they give an unidentifiable hit of umami—savoriness that enhances everything it touches—to all sorts of recipes.

Baking powder: A few of these recipes contain baking powder. The actual leaveners in these do not worry me, but some baking powders contain aluminum, while others have cornstarch, potato starch, or arrowroot. Again, this strikes me as an issue of dose, and it doesn't worry me, but pick which you find most acceptable or skip those recipes.

You can substitute baking soda and cream of tartar for baking powder. One quarter of a teaspoon of baking soda plus ½ teaspoon of cream of tartar is equal to 1 teaspoon of baking powder. (Why the smaller quantity? That's where the cornstarch got left out.) Your body creates bicarbonate of soda, while tartaric acid—cream of tartar—is a natural byproduct of wine production, so this strikes me as quite Paleo. Don't think you can mix this up in quantity and keep it on hand. Without the starchy filler, the baking soda and acid will start to react, leaving you with oomph-less baking powder. You'll just have to add two ingredients instead of one.

Coconut oil spray: I have long made liberal use of nonstick cooking spray, but there's no way it can be considered Paleo. Happily, I found Kelapo Extra Virgin Coconut Oil Cooking Spray at Sahara Mart. It's not essential, but it is useful. If your health food store doesn't carry it, surely they could order it for you. Also, Amazon.com has it.

Broth or stock: I very much hope you will make your own bone broth or stock. It is supremely nutritionally valuable. Still, it is nice to have packaged stock in the house for emergency use. I have used Kitchen Basics brand, which is widely available, and also Costco's Kirkland Organic Chicken Stock. I often reduce these—boil them down by a third or so—to intensify the flavor.

Enjoying This Book

Now that you understand Paleo and my approach to it, let's talk about how to use this book.

What Counts as Five Ingredients?

Each recipe contains five or fewer ingredients. In the interest of giving you tasty, varied food, I have made the executive decision that a few things do not count toward the five ingredient limit: water, salt, pepper, and cooking fats. These will be considered pantry items that you have on hand. Okay? Really, it's all just to give you good recipes.

You'll find that I sometimes suggest possible additions to a recipe, should you feel like taking the extra time and effort. All of the recipes work fine without those additions.

How Were the Nutrition Counts Calculated?

The nutrition counts have been calculated using MasterCook software, a very useful program that allows the user to enter the ingredients of a recipe and the number of servings it makes and then spits out the nutritional breakdown for each serving. MasterCook does not, however, calculate for such things as skimming the fat off of soup or draining and discarding a marinade.

The nutrition counts for these recipes are as accurate as I can make them. However, they cannot be 100 percent accurate. MasterCook gets its nutritional information from the U.S. Department of Agriculture Nutrient Database. MasterCook also lets the user enter new ingredients in the database, and I have done this with ingredients such as coconut aminos and unsweetened coconut milk. In these cases, I have taken the nutritional information from the labels.

Every stalk of celery, slice of onion, and head of broccoli is going to have slightly different levels of vitamins, minerals, and carbohydrate in it because it grew in a specific patch of soil, in specific weather, with a particular kind of fertilizer. Plus, you may use slightly meatier chicken than I do, or you may be a little more or less generous with how many bits of chopped green pepper you fit into a measuring cup, for example.

Don't sweat it. These counts are, as the old joke goes, close enough for government work. The important thing is eating appropriate foods for and skipping the toxic modern interlopers.

Do You Use Microwaves?

I use my microwave all of the time, not just for reheating leftovers, but for cooking, especially for steaming vegetables. I know of no simpler nor more satisfactory method, and my Tupperware microwave steamer is out of the cabinet more often than in it. Further, I have seen some fairly convincing arguments for microwave steaming of vegetables retaining more nutrients than most other cooking methods.

However, I suspect that at least some of the people who read this book will be appalled that I would even consider using a microwave. A faction of them considers microwaves, and all food cooked in them, to be horribly dangerous.

I'm not going to argue the point here. Anything I steam in my microwave, you are welcome to steam on your stovetop. Remember that, technically speaking, all cooking is non-Paleo.

Paleo Staples

This chapter features staples, those ingredients that you keep on hand and draw on often to use in other recipes, such as ketchup, mayonnaise, salad dressing, and seasoning blends. Unfortunately, many of these staples are unavailable in Paleo form because they have sugar, bad oils, or both.

Hence, we have this chapter. These recipes will be called for in *other* recipes. In those recipes, they will count as only one ingredient. That's why this chapter comes first.

Do you have to make all of these? Of course not. It depends on which you feel you'll use often. I generally have on hand homemade ketchup, mayonnaise, two or three kinds of salad dressing, and Creole Seasoning, which I use on everything. Just figure that every few weeks you'll spend an hour or so making your staples, and then you'll have them to draw upon. Really, they're not hard to make. Each of these staples has only five or fewer ingredients, of course.

Dana's Paleo Ketchup

Ketchup is such a fundamental part of American cuisine that we find it hard to do without. Yet everyone's favorite is heavy on the corn syrup. This will serve all ketchup-y purposes, from topping burgers to flavoring meat loaves.

Put everything in a food processor and run the machine until the onion and garlic are pulverized. Pour the mixture into a non-reactive saucepan over medium-low heat, bring the mixture to a simmer, and let it cook for 15 to 20 minutes.

If desired, run it through the food processor again. Store the ketchup in a clean, old jar or a snap-top container in the fridge.

SERVES **12**

1 can (6 ounces, or 190 g) tomato paste

1 can (6 ounces, or 175 ml) water (Fill the tomato paste can with water.)

¼ of a medium onion

½ of a clove of garlic

⅓ cup (80 ml) white balsamic vinegar

2 tablespoons (40 g) honey

½ teaspoon salt

Per serving: 24 calories, trace fat, 1 g protein, 6 g carbohydrate, 1 g dietary fiber, 5 g net carbs

Good Ol' Mayonnaise

Sadly, commercially made mayonnaise is uniformly unPaleo. Even the "made with olive oil" stuff is mostly canola oil.

Put the egg and the yolk in a blender or food processor, along with the vinegar or lemon juice, mustard, and salt.

Measure the oil in a measuring cup with a pouring lip. Turn on the blender or food processor. With it running, pour in the oil in a stream no bigger than a pencil lead in diameter. When it's all in, you're done!

Store the mayonnaise in a tightly lidded jar or snap-top container in the fridge. Use it like any mayonnaise.

SERVES **12**

1 egg plus 1 yolk

2 teaspoons wine vinegar or lemon juice

½ teaspoon dry mustard

¼ teaspoon salt

1 cup (235 ml) MCT oil or light olive oil

2 drops of plain liquid stevia extract, optional

Per serving: 171 calories, 19 g fat, 1 g protein, trace carbohydrate, 0 grams fiber, trace net carbs

notes

You can use extra-virgin olive oil for mayonnaise if you like, but the flavor will be quite strong. You can also use part avocado oil.

A few drops of Frank's Hot Sauce or a few grains of cayenne—not enough to make it hot, just enough for a little accent—would be a classical addition to this, but it's hardly essential.

Balsamic Vinaigrette

This is a great all-around salad dressing for any sort of green salad. It's also good for marinating chicken.

Just measure everything into a clean jar, screw the lid on tight, and shake hard. Store in the fridge and re-shake before using.

SERVES 6

¼ cup (60 ml) balsamic vinegar

½ cup (120 ml) extra-virgin olive oil

2 tablespoons (30 g) spicy brown mustard

1 clove of garlic, crushed

⅛ teaspoon salt

⅛ teaspoon ground black pepper

Per serving: 166 calories, 18 g fat, trace protein, 1 g carbohydrate, trace dietary fiber, 1 g net carbs

White Balsamic Vinaigrette Dressing

Milder than dressing made with red balsamic vinegar, this is great for spring mix and other delicate greens and for any salad, including fruit. I use this stuff all of the time!

Put all of the ingredients in a jar, lid it tightly, and shake like mad!

note

You can change the entire aspect of this dressing by adding ½ teaspoon orange zest and a few drops of orange extract.

SERVES 9

½ cup (120 ml) extra-virgin olive oil, avocado oil, or a combination

⅓ cup (80 ml) white balsamic vinegar

1 clove garlic

½ teaspoon dry mustard

Pinch each of salt and ground black pepper

Per serving: 108 calories, 12 g fat, trace protein, 1 g carbohydrate, trace dietary fiber, 1 g net carbs

Italian Vinaigrette

This may be the most popular dressing in the Western world. You can use this with Greek food, too, or anything Mediterranean.

Put everything in a clean jar, screw the lid on tight, and shake. That's it!

SERVES 6

½ cup (120 ml) extra-virgin olive oil

¼ cup (60 ml) red wine vinegar

1 clove of garlic, crushed

1 teaspoon Italian seasoning

¼ teaspoon salt

⅛ teaspoon ground black pepper

Per serving: 162 calories, 18 g fat, trace protein, 1 g carbohydrate, trace dietary fiber, 1 g net carbs

Apple-y Dressing

I wanted a dressing that really pointed up the apple flavor of apple cider vinegar. This worked beautifully; it's become a staple in my kitchen, both for salads and for cooking. It's great on lettuce, of course, but also on spinach salad with bacon and on Caulirice salads. Or use it to baste pork chops or chicken. This dressing is great freshly made, but the flavors blend more on standing, as the onion infuses into the dressing.

Just put all of the ingredients in a jar, lid it tightly, and shake it hard.

SERVES 6

¼ cup (60 ml) apple cider vinegar

½ cup (120 ml) avocado oil

2 teaspoons spicy brown mustard

2 tablespoons (20 g) minced red onion

Liquid stevia extract, to equal 2 teaspoons (8 g) sugar

Per serving: 165 calories, 18 g fat, trace protein, 1 g carbohydrate, trace dietary fiber, 1 g net carbs

Honey Mustard Dressing and Dipping Sauce

Here's everybody's favorite dipping sauce! It's great for salads, too.

In a bowl, just mix everything together well. This is dipping texture; feel free to thin it a little with water if you want a pourable consistency. Store it in a tightly lidded jar in the fridge.

1 cup (240 ml) Good Ol' Mayonnaise (See page 30.)

¼ cup (60 g) spicy brown mustard

2 tablespoons (40 g) honey

36 drops liquid stevia extract, or to equal 2 tablespoons (26 g) sugar in sweetness

2 tablespoons (30 ml) lemon juice

Per serving: 354 calories, 38 g fat, 1 g protein, 8 g carbohydrate, trace dietary fiber, 8 g net carbs

Basic Stir-Fry Sauce

Any time you need a quick meal, dice up some chicken, pork, or beef or grab a handful of shrimp, whatever you like, and a couple of vegetables, stir-fry them, add the sauce, and dinner is served. If you'd rather not use sherry, you can sub white wine vinegar.

In a bowl, just mix it all together and store in a tightly lidded container in the fridge.

1 cup (235 ml) coconut aminos

4 cloves of garlic, crushed

¼ cup (60 ml) dry sherry

1 tablespoon (8 g) grated ginger root

2 teaspoons dark sesame oil

Per serving: 51 calories, 1 g fat, trace protein, 7 g carbohydrate, trace dietary fiber, 7 g net carbs

note

If you like your stir-fry spicy, sriracha would be the logical hot sauce to add.

Lemon Stir-Fry Sauce

SERVES 8

Throw a few handfuls of shrimp or scallops in a wok or skillet along with some vegetables and boom *supper is served. This sauce is also good over simple steamed fish and in chicken stir-fries.*

To free up the juice, roll both lemons firmly under the heel of your hand. Grate 2 teaspoons lemon zest and then whack the lemons in half and squeeze out every drop of juice into a bowl. Use a spoon to scrape the last bit of juice out of the pulp.

Mix the zest and juice with the rest of the ingredients. Store the sauce in a tightly lidded jar in the fridge.

2 lemons, at room temperature or a bit warmer (Warm citrus yields more juice.)

½ cup (120 ml) chicken broth

3 tablespoons (45 ml) coconut aminos

36 drops of plain liquid stevia extract, to equal 2 tablespoons (26 g) sugar

1 clove of garlic, crushed

Per serving: 11 calories, trace fat, trace protein, 3 g carbohydrate, trace dietary fiber, 3 g net carbs

note

Feel free to add some red pepper flakes or sriracha to this sauce.

Anchovy-Walnut Pesto

SERVES 24

If you love pesto, but shun dairy, you must try this! The anchovies add just the right note of salty umami.

Put the garlic in your food processor and pulse it a few times. Add the basil, walnuts, and anchovies. Turn on the processor and pour the olive oil in through the feed tube. When you have an even paste, stop.

Scrape the pesto into a clean jar. To keep the basil from turning color, you can pour an extra ⅛ inch (3 mm) or so of olive oil on top or smooth a layer of plastic wrap directly on the surface of the pesto. Either way, lid the jar and refrigerate it if you're going to use it up quickly or freeze it if you plan to keep it for a while.

3 cloves of garlic

2 cups (48 g) loosely packed basil leaves

1 cup (100 g) walnuts

2 ounces (55 g) canned anchovies in olive oil, drained

1 cup (235 ml) extra-virgin olive oil

Per serving: 117 calories, 12 g fat, 2 g protein, 1 g carbohydrate, trace dietary fiber, 1 g net carbs

Creole Seasoning

SERVES 48

Creole seasonings such as Tony Chachere's are tremendously versatile. However, Tony Chachere's contains silicon dioxide as an anti-caking agent. Some Paleo folks shun it, but others figure silica is a nutrient. If you make your own, use high-quality salt. Do use good quality, hot paprika here to make up for the lack of cayenne.

Throw everything in a food processor and run it till the celery seed is pulverized, about 2 minutes. Store the mix in a spice shaker.

2 tablespoons (12 g) ground black pepper

⅓ cup (91 g) salt

3 tablespoons (27 g) garlic powder

3 tablespoons (21 g) hot paprika

2 tablespoons (14 g) onion powder

1 tablespoon (6 g) Italian seasoning

2 teaspoons celery seed

Per serving: 5 calories, trace fat, trace protein, 1 g carbohydrate, trace dietary fiber, 1 g net carbs

note

Without the silicon dioxide, this is prone to caking. So save those little desiccant sachets that come in vitamin bottles and the like. They're actually full of silicon dioxide. Bake a used sachet at your oven's lowest temperature for 10 minutes or so to dry it out and then drop it in the shaker. Keep the shaker tightly closed.

Seasoned Salt

SERVES 30

Most commercial seasoned salt contains both sugar and corn-starch. I'm pretty sure you don't want to eat those. This is a snap to stir up, and it will come in handy in all sorts of recipes.

Mix all of the ingredients together and store it in a spice shaker.

½ cup (136 g) salt

2 teaspoons paprika

1 teaspoon turmeric

1 teaspoon garlic powder

1 teaspoon onion powder

Per serving: 1 calorie, trace fat, trace protein, trace carbohydrate, trace dietary fiber, trace net carbs

note

A 50/50 blend of this and Magic Dust (see page 168) is great stuff. However, if you prefer, Real Salt brand makes a good, junk-free seasoned salt. Look for it at your health food store.

Meat Tenderizer

Tough cuts of meat are a nutrition bargain. The connective tissue in them is full of gelatin. Tenderizer can make them more appealing. Sadly, I can no longer find meat tenderizer that contains no junk. However, thanks to Amazon.com, I obtained more papain—which is the papaya enzyme that has been used as a tenderizer for a very long time—than I can possibly use in a lifetime. Use this mixture as you would a commercial meat tenderizer. (You can't use straight papain as you would commercial meat tenderizer or you will end up with meat porridge. It's strong stuff. That's why we're mixing it with other ingredients.)

Stir the seasoned salt together with the papain, making sure it's completely blended. Store in a tightly lidded old spice shaker.

½ cup (150 g) Seasoned Salt
(See page 35.) or seasoned salt,
such as Real Salt

2 teaspoons papain enzyme

Per serving: 5 calories, trace fat,
trace protein, 1 g carbohydrate,
trace dietary fiber, 1 g net carbs

notes

You can vary this. I've made a good version using Magic Dust (see page 168), smoked paprika, and papain. You could also use the Creole Seasoning (see page 35). You just need to pay attention to proportions. Papain is powerful stuff; you don't want to make meat porridge. If you want to make just a small batch, go with 1 tablespoon (15 g) seasonings and ¼ teaspoon papain.

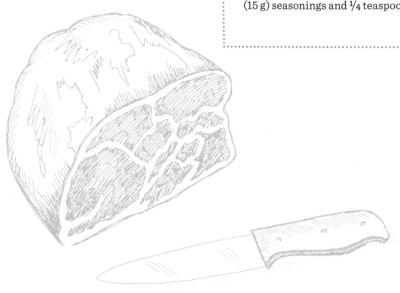

Italian-Seasoned Pork Rind Crumbs

These are great for "breading" pork chops, chicken, or fish.

Run the pork rinds through a food processor until they're crumbs. Add everything else and pulse to combine. Store in a tightly lidded jar in the refrigerator.

3½ ounces (99 g) pork rinds (one average bag)

1 teaspoon Italian seasoning

¼ teaspoon garlic powder

¼ teaspoon onion powder

Per serving: 91 calories, 5 g fat, 10 g protein, trace carbohydrate, trace dietary fiber, 0 g net carbs

Coconut Sour Cream

For those of you who are dairy free, you can culture coconut milk or coconut cream to make Coconut Sour Cream.

Refrigerate the can of coconut milk overnight. In the morning, open the can and scoop off the thick cream that will have risen to the top. Place it in a snap-top container or jar and stir in the contents of the probiotic capsule. Put in a warm place; I use an old electric hot pad for this purpose, tuck it down in a bowl, and set it on low. Let it sit overnight and then refrigerate. Use just as you would sour cream (or yogurt).

Sometimes this separates. You can stir it up, or you can pour off the liquid.

1 can (14 ounces, or 390 ml) unsweetened coconut milk

Contents of a probiotic capsule (I use one with 10 different strains that I buy from Puritan's Pride.)

Per serving: It depends upon the brand of coconut milk.

Snacks, Nibbles, and Party Foods

This chapter is about the stuff you eat with your hands, the stuff you can put out when friends come over to see the big game, on movie night, or for impromptu celebrations. Everybody loves finger food!

These foods are also great to have in the refrigerator or pantry for those moments when you need something to eat *right now!* With a few of these on hand, the chances that you'll resort to eating junk are dramatically reduced.

About Wings

A few of the recipes in this chapter are wing sauces. Everybody loves wings, and you'll have a bounty of bones for your next pot of broth. Sadly, restaurant hot wings are usually floured or breaded and fried in questionable fat. It's so unnecessary! You can grill your wings or roast them, just get 'em good and crisp. The serving count assumes cut-up wings. If you've got whole wings, which are less work, obviously, figure that the sauce will coat a dozen. The nutrition counts are for the sauce only, not for the wings.

Addictive Punks

Omigosh. Make a batch of these on family video night and serve them warm. No one will miss the popcorn!

Preheat the oven to 350°F (180°C or gas mark 4).

Put the bacon grease in a big, shallow roasting pan and stick it in the oven while it's heating. When the bacon grease has melted, add the pumpkin seeds and stir them around till they're all coated. Spread them out and bake them for 5 minutes. Stir the pumpkin seeds, spread them out again, and bake them for another 5 minutes.

In the meanwhile, in a small bowl, stir the seasonings together.

When the timer beeps again, pull out your now lovely, toasty seeds and sprinkle the seasoning mixture over them. Sprinkle a bit, stir a bit, sprinkle a bit, and stir a bit to get them evenly coated. Serve warm, though they're awfully good after they cool, too.

SERVES 8

1 tablespoon (14 g) bacon grease

2 cups (454 g) shelled pumpkin seeds, a.k.a. pepitas

½ teaspoon onion powder

½ teaspoon garlic powder

½ teaspoon paprika (I used hot, but do as you like.)

1½ teaspoons salt

Per serving: 312 calories, 26 g fat, 19 g protein, 8 g carbohydrate, 2 g dietary fiber, 6 g net carbs

Dirty Punks

Pumpkin and squash seeds are as nutritious as they are delicious. It's the caramelized juice that makes these special.

Preheat the oven to 350°F (180°C or gas mark 4).

Scoop the seeds out of the pumpkin or squash. Do not rinse them! You don't even have to remove every bit of the strings; a little bit of string clinging to the seeds just improves them. Spread them in a shallow metal baking sheet. (I use my jelly roll pan.)

In a medium bowl, stir together about 1 teaspoon of oil or fat for every 1 cup (64 g) of seeds till all of the seeds are coated. Spread them in a single layer in the pan.

Roast the seeds for 10 minutes and then stir. Roast the seeds for another 10 minutes, stir again, and give them a final 10 minutes. Salt the seeds lightly and eat immediately!

YIELD VARIES

Seeds fresh from a pumpkin or other winter squash, such as butternut, acorn, Hubbard, or spaghetti

Coconut oil, bacon grease, or lard

Salt

Per serving: It depends upon the amount of seeds used.

Sriracha Punks

Hot and garlicky, these will be the hit of your next party, especially if you serve them warm. Try them sprinkled over a salad, too.

Preheat the oven to 350°F (180°C or gas mark 4).

In the meantime, spread the pumpkin seeds on a shallow rimmed baking sheet. Drizzle the sriracha evenly over the seeds. Using a rubber scraper, stir the seeds until they're all evenly coated.

In a small bowl, stir together the garlic powder and salt. Sprinkle the mixture evenly over the seeds and again stir till they're all evenly coated.

Spread the seeds out in an even layer and stick 'em in the oven. Bake the seeds for 5 minutes. Then stir them, spread them out again, and bake them for another 5 minutes.

At this point, check to see whether they're dry. (You want the sriracha to have dried on the seeds.) If they're dry, pull 'em out. If they're still a bit damp, stir them one more time and give them another few minutes.

When your seeds are done, take a look: Is the salt and garlic mixture adhering to your seeds? Or is it lying on the bottom of the pan? If the salt refuses to stick, stir in the oil while the seeds are still hot, again coating evenly. The salt will adhere nicely.

Serve immediately or store in a snap-top container.

2 cups (450 g) shelled pumpkin seeds, aka pepitas

2 tablespoons (30 ml) sriracha

½ teaspoon garlic powder

1 teaspoon salt

1 teaspoon coconut oil (optional)

Per serving: 302 calories, 24 g fat, 19 g protein, 8 g carbohydrate, 2 g dietary fiber, 6 g net carbs

Bacon 'n Eggs

When I discovered that Koop's brand horseradish mustard had no junk in it, creating this recipe was my very first thought. I took these to my Toastmasters Christmas party, and they promptly evaporated.

This is your basic Deviled Egg procedure: Peel the eggs. Halve them, turning the yolks into a bowl. Add the mayonnaise and horseradish mustard and mash 'em up really well. (I start with a fork, and then I use the back of a big spoon to mash any lumps against the side of the bowl.)

When the yolk mixture is creamy, spoon or pipe it into the whites. Crumble the bacon and sprinkle a little over each egg.

SERVES 12

6 eggs, hard-boiled

¼ cup (60 g) Good Ol' Mayonnaise (See page 30.)

1 tablespoon (15 g) horseradish mustard

2 slices of cooked bacon (I leave it up to you how it gets cooked; just see that it's crisp.)

Per serving: 79 calories, 7 g fat, 4 g protein, trace carbohydrate, trace dietary fiber, 0 g net carbs

Eggs in Tunisia

Harissa is an exotic seasoning paste from Northern Africa. I loved it instantly, but when I read labels, I discovered that a lot of harissa has sugar and other objectionable ingredients. As mentioned earlier, I use Mina brand harissa—no sugar!

You know the drill: Peel the eggs and then halve them, turning the yolks into a mixing bowl. Add everything else and smash it all up, till the yolks are smooth and creamy. Pipe or spoon the mixture back into the whites.

SERVES 12

6 eggs, hard-boiled

¼ cup (60 g) Good Ol' Mayonnaise (See page 30.)

2 tablespoons (32 g) harissa

1 small clove of garlic or ½ of a large clove of garlic, crushed

¼ teaspoon cumin

¼ teaspoon salt

Per serving: 74 calories, 7 g fat, 3 g protein, 1 g carbohydrate, trace dietary fiber, 1 g net carbs

Sriracha Eggs

SERVES
12

These are deviled eggs with a hot and spicy Southeast Asian twist.

Peel the eggs, halve 'em, and turn the yolks out into a mixing bowl. Add everything but the cilantro to the yolks and mash it all up until it's creamy. Spoon or pipe the mixture back into the whites.

Just before serving, sprinkle a little cilantro over each egg. If you're a cilantro-hater, then skip it. They'll still be yummy.

6 eggs, hard-boiled

¼ cup (60 g) Good Ol' Mayonnaise (See page 30.)

1 tablespoon (15 ml) sriracha

½ teaspoon fish sauce

2 tablespoons (32 g) minced cilantro (optional)

Per serving: 72 calories, 7 g fat, 3 g protein, trace carbohydrate, trace dietary fiber, 0 g net carbs

Egg Yolk Dip

SERVES
4

I came up with this when I made the Biscuits on page 48 for the first time. As I separated the eggs, I slipped the yolks into simmering water. When they were done, I made this. If you love deviled eggs, this is for you.

In a bowl, mash the yolks thoroughly.

Mince the scallions fine and add to the yolks along with everything else. Stir and mash until the mixture is smooth.

I used celery with this dip, but peppers would be good, too. Or you could spread it on the biscuits!

4 egg yolks

2 scallions

¼ cup (60 g) Good Ol' Mayonnaise (See page 30.)

2 teaspoons whole-grain Dijon mustard

¼ teaspoon salt

2 pinches of ground black pepper

Per serving: 162 calories, 17 g fat, 3 g protein, 1 g carbohydrate, trace dietary fiber, 1 g net carb

Rumaki

These were one of the hot party foods when I was a kid, and surely that was back during the Ice Age. They're delicious, and the fact that they will get some liver into your family is reason enough to make 'em.

Chicken livers sort of naturally divide into two lobes; cut them apart there. Keep your eye out for any black or dark green spots. Those are bile, and while it's not harmful, it is the bitterest substance on Earth. So if you see it, cut it out! Drop the livers in a bowl as you cut 'em up.

Pour in the Basic Stir-Fry Sauce, which I'm figuring you keep on hand, because, geez, it's useful. Stir it up. Now let the livers soak for at least 20 to 30 minutes.

Okay, it's assembly time! I sprayed my broiler rack with coconut oil cooking spray, but it's not essential. Grab some sturdy toothpicks. (Some people soak their toothpicks in water for 30 minutes before assembling these. I didn't, and I had no problems, but feel free to soak yours if you wish.) Turn on the broiler to heat and arrange the oven rack about 8 inches (20 cm) away.

Take a piece of liver. Wrap it, as much as it will wrap, around a water chestnut chunk. Wrap a strip of bacon securely around that and impale the whole thing with a toothpick, taking care to stab it through both the liver and the water chestnut. Arrange 'em on the broiler rack as you go. Repeat until you run out of something.

Now broil the bundles, using tongs to turn and rearrange them as needed, until the bacon is crisp. Serve hot. Fabulous!

12 ounces (340 g) chicken livers

¼ cup (60 ml) Basic Stir-Fry Sauce (See page 33.)

4 ounces (115 g) canned water chestnuts, halved (If you can get fresh water chestnuts, use them! They're not easy to find.)

1½ pounds (680 g) bacon

Per serving: 186 calories, 15 g fat, 11 g protein, 2 g carbohydrate, trace dietary fiber, 2 g net carbs

notes

I can't guarantee that your amount of livers, bacon, and water chestnuts will come out even; that's just the nature of these things. Sorry.

I tried wrapping each liver-and-water-chestnut bundle in a half slice of bacon. Believe me, a whole slice is better.

Brandied Pâté

Add the superior nutrition of liver to your diet in gourmet fashion—and with only a few minutes of work. Stuff this into celery, put it in omelets, or spread it on Paleo crackers.

Heat a medium nonstick skillet over medium-low heat, melt 1 tablespoon (14 g) of the bacon grease, and sauté the shallot until soft. Transfer the shallot to a food processor.

Snip the chicken livers into bite-sized bits.

When the shallot is in the food processor, put the skillet back over the heat. Melt the remaining 1 tablespoon (14 g) bacon grease and throw in the liver bits. Sauté the liver, turning it frequently, until just barely done. (The largest piece should still be pink in the center.)

Add the cognac, stir, and pour in any juice left from the livers. Let it cook down for a minute or two. Transfer it to your food processor.

Now run the food processor till the whole thing is smooth and creamy. Add the salt and pepper and process till they're evenly worked in. Taste, adjust seasoning if needed, and then scrape into a ramekin or bowl. Chill until set.

Pâté Stuffed Mushrooms

Because the pâté has only four ingredients, this has five!

Preheat the oven to 350°F (180°C or gas mark 4).

Take the pâté out of the fridge to get the chill off.

Remove the stems from the mushrooms, saving them for making omelets or something. Arrange them in a roasting pan and brush them with the bacon grease on both sides.

Bake for 20 to 25 minutes or until soft. Stuff 'em with the pâté and serve! That's it.

SERVES 8

2 tablespoons (28 g) bacon grease, divided

1 small shallot, minced

6 ounces (170 g) chicken livers

1 tablespoon (15 ml) cognac

¼ teaspoon salt, or to taste

⅛ teaspoon ground black pepper, or to taste

Per serving: 82 calories, 5 g fat, 5 g protein, 1 g carbohydrate, trace dietary fiber, 0 g net carbs

SERVES 15

Brandied Pâté (See recipe above.)

8 ounces (225 g) mushrooms

¼ cup (55 g) bacon grease, melted

Per mushroom: 68 calories, 6 g fat, 2 g protein, 1 g carbohydrate, trace dietary fiber, 1 g net carbs

note

If you're going to add an ingredient, I'd make it a little minced parsley or chives, for contrast.

Tripoli Wings

Are you bored with Buffalo Wings? Try these hot wings, which are made with the flavors of North Africa. They're spicy, but not blow-the-top-of-your-head-off hot. Look for Mina brand harissa because it has no sugar. Roast the wings till they're good and crispy. I'd do 'em at 400°F (200°C or gas mark 6) for about 20 to 25 minutes.

Mix the oil, lemon juice, and harissa together in a big, nonreactive bowl. Toss the sauce over the cooked wings.

SERVES 24

¼ cup (60 ml) extra-virgin olive oil

2 tablespoons (28 ml) lemon juice

2 teaspoons harissa

Per serving: 21 calories, 2 g fat, trace protein, trace carbohydrate, trace dietary fiber, 0 g net carbs

Chipotle Wing Sauce

The smoky-hot flavor of chipotle peppers has taken the country by storm. If you'd rather skip the honey, you could increase the liquid stevia instead. Or you could use sugar-free imitation honey. That's what I did. Roast your wings till they're good and crispy. I'd do 'em at 400°F (200°C or gas mark 6) for about 20 to 25 minutes.

Mix the hot sauce, vinegar, butter or fat, honey, and stevia together in a big, nonreactive bowl. Toss the sauce over the cooked wings.

SERVES 24

¼ cup (60 ml) Melinda's chipotle hot sauce

¼ cup (60 ml) cider vinegar

¼ cup (55 g) butter or fat of choice

2 tablespoons (40 g) honey

Liquid stevia extract to equal 1 tablespoon (13 g) sugar

Per serving: 23 calories, 2 g fat, trace protein, 2 g carbohydrate, trace dietary fiber, 2 g net carbs

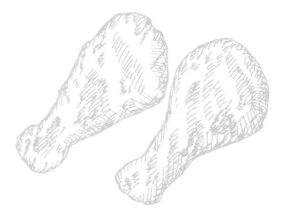

Quasi-Southeast-Asian Wing Sauce

Not authentic, but awfully good, this wing sauce has a Vietnamese sort of accent. Once again, I think minced cilantro would be good here. Toss this sauce with crispy hot wings, either grilled or roasted.

In a medium bowl, just stir it all up.

SERVES 24

2 tablespoons (28 ml) fish sauce

2 tablespoons (28 ml) white balsamic vinegar

2 tablespoons (28 ml) lime juice

1 clove of garlic, crushed

Liquid stevia extract to equal 2 teaspoons sugar or to taste

Per serving: 2 calories, trace fat, trace protein, trace carbohydrate, trace dietary fiber, 0 g net carbs

Chicken Chips

These are awfully good and seriously Paleo. Ask your specialty butcher to save chicken skins for you—you know, from the chicken they skin for all those poor chumps who think it's bad for them.

Preheat the oven to 350°F (180°C or gas mark 4).

Place the skin flat on your broiler rack. Bake for 20 to 25 minutes until crisp. Salt them and stuff in your face. Repeat. We have been known to have just chicken chips for supper!

YIELD VARIES

Chicken skins

Salt, to taste

Per serving: It depends upon the amount of chicken skins and how crispy they are roasted.

A Few Grain-Like Things

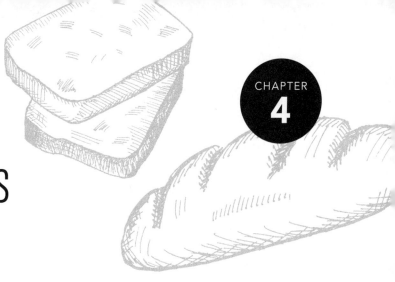

I have only a few, as you can see. Paleo breads are an interesting proposition, generally involving considerably more than five ingredients. They also often include ingredients I won't use or ingredients I don't consider Paleo, such as arrowroot, which is both a concentrated, refined carb and from a plant that has to be processed to be edible. Here are a few bready items, plus a couple of "cereals," one hot and the other cold.

Biscuits

SERVES
6

This is my take on a recipe that originated with Sarah, of the Primitive Palate. *She used coconut oil in her biscuits, but I liked the idea of lard, and bacon grease would be good, too. I came up with the muffin tin idea, too, and a good idea it was. It gives them a nice shape. These are very rich and therefore very filling. Serve them hot with butter.*

Preheat the oven to 350°F (180°C or gas mark 4). Grease a six-muffin tin well with lard or coconut oil or use coconut oil cooking spray. (I did this even though my muffin tin was non-stick, and I recommend you do the same.)

About those egg whites: Be sure there's not the teeniest speck of yolk in them. If there's even a pinhead's worth, they will stubbornly refuse to whip. The same is true if there's any grease at all on the bowl or beaters. It's worth washing and drying them again, just to be sure. Now, whip the egg whites until they're stiff.

Put the rest of the ingredients in your food processor with the S-blade in place. Pulse until the lard is thoroughly cut into the almond meal.

Grab a rubber scraper. Sprinkle about ¼ cup (35 g) of the almond meal mixture over the egg whites and gently fold it in. Repeat, working gently and gingerly, until all the almond meal mixture is folded in. (Do be gentle because the bubbles are what make the biscuits light.)

Using an ice cream scoop, scoop the batter into the prepared muffin tins, filling the cups evenly. (If you don't have a scoop, use a spoon.) Bake for 20 minutes. Yum.

4 egg whites, at room temperature

1½ cups (168 g) almond meal

⅓ cup (75 g) lard

1 teaspoon baking powder

½ teaspoon salt

Per serving: 255 calories, 18 g fat, 16 g protein, 10 g carbohydrate, 0 g dietary fiber, 10 g net carbs

note

Don't you dare throw away the egg yolks! Make the Egg Yolk Dip on page 42 or one of the custards in the Desserts chapter. Or just scramble them into your breakfast. But wasting egg yolks is a terrible thing. They're where all the vitamins and antioxidants are.

Coconut Flax Bread

This bread is great toasted and buttered! It's even better if you add some of the Brandied Pâté on page 44. Or toast it and enjoy it with pâté and a fried egg on top! The possibilities are endless. This will not rise up as high as wheat-based yeast bread. I considered increasing the volume of all the ingredients, but I worried about the edges overcooking before the middle was done. Just have two slices. Or, heck, have three.

Preheat the oven to 350°F (180°C or gas mark 4). Line a loaf pan with nonstick foil. (Reynolds makes this. You could use baking parchment if you prefer, but nonstick foil is da bomb.)

Put the coconut in a food processor with the S-blade in place and run it for 5 to 7 minutes, stopping now and then to scrape down the sides. Add the flaxseed meal, salt, and baking soda and pulse till they're well mixed in, again, scraping down the sides if you need to. With the processor running, add the eggs, one at a time, letting each one blend in before adding another. When 4 of the eggs are in, add the vinegar. Add the final 2 eggs, one at a time.

Scrape the batter into the prepared pan. Bake for 45 to 50 minutes till golden and pulling away from the sides of the pan. Turn out of the pan and cool on a wire rack.

Store in a sealed zipper-lock bag in the refrigerator. This slices best with a thin, straight-bladed knife.

2 cups (160 g) shredded coconut

½ cup (56 g) flaxseed meal

½ teaspoon salt

1 teaspoon baking soda

6 eggs

1 tablespoon (15 ml) vinegar

Per serving: 101 calories, 8 g fat, 4 g protein, 4 g carbohydrate, 3 g dietary fiber, 1 g net carbs

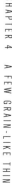

CHAPTER 4 A FEW GRAIN-LIKE THINGS

49

Porky-Pumpy-Pie-Pancakes

SERVES
6

Yes, these are really good. And if you don't tell people they have pork rinds in them, they will never guess. By the way, pork rinds are health food. They are a great source of gelatin. Serve these pancakes with butter and a drop or two of syrup or honey, if you insist.

There's nothing tricky here. Just put everything in a bowl and whisk it up. Let it sit for 5 minutes to thicken. You might as well get a skillet or griddle heating in the meantime.

When the 5 minutes are up, the batter will have thickened quite a bit. Add water to thin the batter to your preference. (I used about ⅓ cup [80 ml]. I like 'em thick.) Fry like you would any pancakes.

1 cup (245 g) canned pumpkin

1½ ounces (43 g) pork rinds, ground to crumbs in your food processor

6 eggs

½ teaspoon English toffee–flavored liquid stevia extract, or more, to taste

2 teaspoons pumpkin pie spice

Per serving: 159 calories, 9 g fat, 15 g protein, 4 g carbohydrate, 1 g dietary fiber, 3 g net carbs

Primal Pancakes and Waffles

SERVES
8

Cream cheese pancakes are popular among low carbers, but I couldn't find additive-free cream cheese, not even at the health food store. Mascarpone is cleaner, and it works beautifully! Maple syrup is okay, if you can deal with the carbs. Pureed, lightly sweetened berries are good, as is erythritol with a little cinnamon stirred in.

Start by putting a skillet or griddle on a medium burner or plugging in a waffle iron. (You want it hot when your batter is ready.)

Just put everything in a blender and run it, scraping down the sides once or twice, until it's evenly mixed. Cook like any normal pancakes or waffles.

4 ounces (115 g) mascarpone cheese

4 eggs

⅓ cup (37 g) almond meal

½ teaspoon salt

½ teaspoon baking powder

6 drops of English toffee– or vanilla-flavored liquid stevia extract

---

Per serving: 120 calories, 10 g fat, 6 g protein, 3 g carbohydrate, 0 g dietary fiber, 3 g net carbs

Coconut Maple-Cinnamon Flakes

SERVES
8

These make a great substitute for cold cereal. Eat with coconut milk, milk, cream, or sprinkled over yogurt.

Preheat the oven to 325°F (170°C or gas mark 3). Line your large, shallow baking sheet with foil.

Place the coconut in a large mixing bowl. Add the salt, cinnamon, stevia, and vanilla extract and stir until the salt is dissolved.

Sprinkle the water over the coconut mixture 1 tablespoon (15 ml) at a time, mixing very thoroughly after each addition. (You want to wind up with all the coconut flakes evenly coated with the water mixture.) Now, again, 1 tablespoon (20 ml) at a time, stir in the maple syrup, stirring after each addition, till all the coconut is evenly coated.

Spread the coconut in an even layer in the prepared pan. Bake for 15 minutes and then stir everything carefully but well and spread it out evenly again.

Continue baking for another 10 to 15 minutes, stirring every 5 minutes, until the flakes are evenly golden. (Don't neglect to stir every 5 minutes! The oven timer is your friend.)

Allow the flakes to cool and store in a snap-top container.

4 cups (240 g) flaked coconut

½ teaspoon salt

½ teaspoon cinnamon

¼ teaspoon English toffee–flavored liquid stevia extract

1 teaspoon vanilla extract

¼ cup (60 ml) water

¼ cup (80 g) maple syrup

Per serving: 168 calories, 13 g fat, 1 g protein, 13 g carbohydrate, 4 g dietary fiber, 9 g net carbs

note

To drop the carb count, swap ¼ cup (48 g) erythritol plus ⅛ teaspoon real maple extract for the maple syrup. Mix the maple extract with the water and then sprinkle on the erythritol, stirring constantly, once the coconut is evenly dampened. Keep in mind that because of the reduced liquid content, this will toast faster.

Toasted Almond and Coconut "Cereal"

Warm and comforting, the toasting of the almond and coconut in this "cereal" deepens the flavor. I loved Wheatena in my youth, and this reminds me of it—only with no gluten, of course.

Preheat the oven to 350°F (180°C or gas mark 4).

In a bowl, mix the coconut and almond meal and spread it in a large roasting pan. Toast for 2 minutes, stir, and then toast for another 2 to 3 minutes, just until golden.

In the roasting pan, mix the toasted coconut and almond meal with the flaxseed meal and chia seeds. Store in a snap-top container in the fridge.

To serve, put ⅓ cup (35 g) of the mixture in a small bowl, stir in a small pinch of salt, and add ¾ cup (175 ml) boiling water. Stir and then cover with a saucer and let soak for 5 minutes. Eat like any cold cereal.

SERVES
12

1½ cups (120 g) shredded coconut

1½ cups (168 g) almond meal

¾ cup (84 g) flaxseed meal

¼ cup (52 g) chia seeds

Salt

Per serving: 198 calories, 13 g fat, 11 g protein, 13 g carbohydrate, 7 g dietary fiber, 6 g net carbs

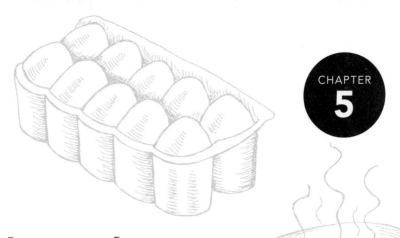

Eggs

All you need to know about my relationship with eggs can be summarized thusly: As I write this, there are thirty chickens running around my yard. Thirty. Eggs are not only wildly nutritious, they are also infinitely variable, both in the ways you can cook them and in the ways they combine with other foods.

Eggs are also, of course, Paleo. Our ancestors ate a wide variety of eggs, from birds and also from reptiles, fish, and insects. After all, eggs don't run or fight back. I'm not suggesting you eat termite caviar, but if your local farmers' market has duck, quail, or turkey eggs, you might grab them for a treat.

If at all possible, pop for pasture-raised eggs. "Cage-free" and "free range" are not the same; the chickens are still inside, not outdoors eating grass, clover, worms, and bugs. Speaking of worms and bugs, don't pay an extra dime for eggs from "chickens fed all-vegetarian feed." Chickens don't like that. They're little dinosaurs, and they love animal food, whether it's bugs, baby snakes and toads, kitchen scraps and refrigerator dregs, or ticks. Yes, chickens turn ticks into eggs. Beat that magic trick.

If you've never had fresh eggs from chickens allowed to run outside and scratch in the lawn, you will be dazzled by the way the whites stand up plump around the rich, orange yolks. You'll never go back.

I will start with perhaps my most-repeated bit of cookery instruction.

Dana's Easy Omelet Method

If I had to choose just one skill to teach to everyone trying to improve his or her diet, it would be how to make an omelet. They're fast, they're easy, and they make a wide variety of simple ingredients seem like a meal!

First, have your filling ready. If you're using vegetables, sauté them first. If you're making an omelet to use up leftovers, a great idea by the way, warm them through in the microwave and have them standing by.

The pan matters here. For omelets, I recommend an 8- to 9-inch (20 to 23 cm) nonstick skillet with sloping sides. Even if you've been nervous about Teflon or Silverstone, take a look at the new ceramic nonstick pans. They're wonderful. Put your skillet over medium-high heat. While the skillet's heating, grab your eggs—two is the perfect number for this size pan, but one or three will work—and a bowl, crack the eggs,

and beat them with a fork. Don't add anything, just mix them up.

The pan is hot enough when a drop of water thrown in sizzles right away. Add a little fat, whatever works with the ingredients of your omelet, and slosh it around to cover the bottom. Now pour in the eggs, all at once. They should sizzle and immediately start to set. When the bottom layer of egg is set around the edges—this should happen quite quickly—lift the edge using a spatula or fork and tip the pan to let the raw egg flow underneath. Do this all around the edges until there's not enough raw egg to run.

Now, turn your burner to the lowest heat if you have a gas stove. If you have an electric stove, you'll need to have a "warm" burner standing by because electric elements don't cool off fast enough for this job. Put your filling on one half of the omelet, cover it, and let it sit over very low heat for a minute or two, no more. Peek and see if the raw, shiny egg is gone from the top surface. (Although you can serve it that way if you like. That's how the French prefer their omelets.)

When your omelet is done, slip a spatula under the half without the filling, fold it over, and then lift the whole thing onto a plate.

This makes a single-serving omelet. I think it's a lot easier to make several individual omelets than to make one big one, and omelets are so quick to make that it's not that big a deal. Anyway, that way you can customize your omelets to each individual's taste. If you're making more than two or three omelets, keep them warm in your oven, set to its very lowest heat.

BAT Omelet

SERVES
1

Hey, what's not to love about bacon, avocados, and tomatoes? If you're eating primal, an ounce (28 g) or so of Monterey Jack cheese would be good here, too. If you use cheese (come to think of it, Queso Quesadilla would be good, too), put it in first, then the avocado, and then the tomato.

First cook your bacon until crisp. Set it aside.

Scramble up the eggs and make the omelet according to Dana's Easy Omelet Method on page 54, layering in the avocado first and then the tomato. Crumble in the bacon just before folding and serve.

2 slices of bacon

2 eggs

½ of an avocado, peeled, pitted, and sliced

1 small tomato, sliced or diced

Per serving: 392 calories, 31 g fat, 18 g protein, 14 g carbohydrate, 4 g dietary fiber, 10 g net carbs

note

I served this with chipotle hot sauce, but you know me, I'd put hot sauce on a hot fudge sundae—not that I'd eat a hot fudge sundae.

Spinach-Avocado-Bacon-Sprout Omelet

SERVES
1

You'll notice a certain similarity to the previous omelet. I couldn't choose between alfalfa sprouts and tomato for my fifth ingredient, so I tried it both ways. They're both wonderful! You could do both, you know.

Make your omelet according to Dana's Easy Omelet Method on page 54, layering in the filling in the order given. Fold, plate, and eat. That's it!w

2 eggs

2 teaspoons bacon grease

¾ cup (23 g) loosely packed fresh spinach

½ of an avocado, peeled, pitted, and sliced

3 slices of cooked bacon, crumbled

¼ cup (8 g) alfalfa sprouts

Per serving: 489 calories, 42 g fat, 20 g protein, 10 g carbohydrate, 3 g dietary fiber, 7 g net carbs

Sardine Omelets

SERVES 2

Sardines have a lot going for them: As little fish, they're far less likely to be contaminated with mercury than big ones. They're high in calcium and omega-3 fatty acids. And they keep, of course, so you can have them on hand when you want something quick and filling.

This is so easy! Drain most of the oil off the sardines, leaving a little for the flavor, and dump 'em in a bowl. Add the sour cream, mustard, coconut aminos, and pepper and use a fork to coarsely mash everything together. Add a little salt if you think it needs it.

Make your omelet according to Dana's Easy Omelet Method on page 54 using two eggs and half the filling for each. Keep the first omelet warm in your oven, set to its lowest temperature, while you make the second. Or just eat in shifts. A sliced scallion would be good here. So would a little snipped parsley, should you have any on hand.

4 ounces (115 g) sardines in olive oil

¼ cup (60 g) sour cream or Coconut Sour Cream (See page 37.)

1 teaspoon spicy brown mustard

½ teaspoon coconut aminos

1 pinch of ground black pepper

Salt (optional)

4 eggs

1 tablespoon (15 ml) olive oil

Per serving: 412 calories, 33 g fat, 26 g protein, 4 g carbohydrate, trace dietary fiber, 4 g net carbs

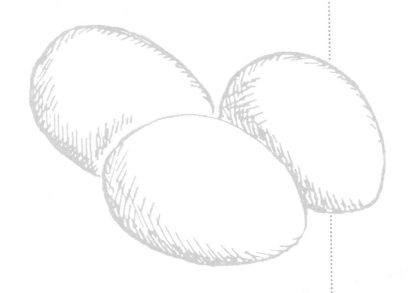

Rumaki Omelet

I was making Rumaki when I thought, "This would make a great omelet!" So I saved some livers and water chestnuts and tried it. I was right. It's a great omelet, and it's very filling.

First put the livers in a small dish or a zipper-lock bag, add the Basic Stir-Fry Sauce, and turn to coat. Let the livers marinate for at least 15 minutes.

Put your omelet-making skillet over medium heat and snip the bacon into it with your kitchen shears. Fry the bits until crispy and then remove them to a plate.

While the bacon is cooking, drain the sauce from the livers, reserving it. Snip the livers into bite-sized bits.

You've got bacon grease left in the skillet, right? Throw in the liver bits and water chestnuts and sauté till the liver has stopped running red. (Don't overcook; the liver should still be a little pink in the middle.) Pour in the reserved sauce, let it simmer for 30 seconds or so, and then remove it.

Give your skillet a wipe if it's sticky. Put it back over the burner, and turn it up to medium high. Melt that extra bacon grease.

Scramble up the eggs and make the omelet according to Dana's Easy Omelet Method on page 54, layering in the chicken liver mixture before you cover the pan. Add the bacon right before folding and serve.

3 chicken livers

2 tablespoons (28 ml) Basic Stir-Fry Sauce (See page 33.)

2 slices of bacon

2 tablespoons (16 g) chopped water chestnut, about 2 water chestnuts

2 eggs

1½ teaspoons bacon grease

Per serving: 426 calories, 26 g fat, 32 g protein, 11 g carbohydrate, trace dietary fiber, 11 g net carbs

Foo Yong-y Omelet

SERVES 1

Tasty, filling, super nutritious, and infinitely variable, this is a great way to use up bits of vegetables kicking around the fridge. You'll notice this does not use Dana's Easy Omelet method, but instead it's cooked all together, Chinese fashion.

As always with Chinese-style cooking, have everything prepped before you start cooking: the mushroom chopped, the scallion sliced, the bean sprouts at hand, and the eggs scrambled.

Put your medium-sized skillet over high heat and melt the lard. Add the mushrooms and scallion and stir-fry for a minute or two, just until the mushrooms start to soften. Add the bean sprouts and stir-fry another minute. Add the Basic Stir-Fry Sauce and stir it in. Spread the vegetables in an even layer covering the bottom of the pan and then pour in the eggs. Tip the pan to spread the egg out over the whole bottom, encompassing all of the vegetables. Turn the burner down to medium-low, cover, and let it cook till set. Flip, if you like, to cook the other side.

Or feel free to do this the easy way, if you prefer, by simply scrambling the eggs with the vegetables.

1 tablespoon (14 g) lard or coconut oil

¼ cup (18 g) chopped mushrooms

1 scallion, sliced

½ cup (26 g) mung bean sprouts

2 teaspoons Basic Stir-Fry Sauce (See page 33.)

2 eggs

Per serving: 283 calories, 22 g fat, 13 g protein, 8 g carbohydrate, 2 g dietary fiber, 6 g net carbs

notes

I used this combination of vegetables because they were cluttering up my fridge. But you can use almost anything you have on hand: thinly sliced onion instead of the scallions, shredded cabbage, snow peas cut into 1-inch (2.5 cm) lengths, thinly sliced celery, and even shredded carrot.

If you have leftover meat in the fridge and are willing to go beyond five ingredients, your horizons broaden still further. Add a handful of cubed leftover chicken, pork, beef, or shrimp, and you've got supper. Feel free to simply double, triple, or quadruple this to feed the whole family.

Shirred Eggs with Bacon, Mushrooms, and Spinach

SERVES
6

You wouldn't make these on a busy weekday morning. But if you ever have a half dozen people over for breakfast and want to be able to set their eggs in front of them all at once, this is the way to go.

Preheat the oven to 350°F (180°C or gas mark 4). Grease six 8-ounce (235 ml) ramekins.

Chop the bacon or use your kitchen shears to snip it into a skillet over medium-low heat. Let it fry a few minutes, stirring and breaking the bits apart. As some of the fat cooks out of the bacon, add the mushrooms. Break them up a bit more with the edge of your spatula as you sauté them with the bacon.

When the bacon is about ⅔ cooked, assemble your eggs: Put a big handful of spinach in each ramekin. It'll cook down, so fill them about ⅔ of the way. Divide the mushroom-bacon mixture among the ramekins, spooning it on top of the spinach. Break an egg into each dish, taking care not to break the yolks. Drizzle a teaspoon of coconut milk or cream on top of each egg.

You can put the ramekins into your roasting pan for easier handling, if you like. Stick 'em all in the oven. Bake for 15 minutes until the whites are set but the yolks are still runny. Serve immediately!

8 slices of bacon

8 ounces (22 g) sliced mushrooms

10 ounces (280 g) fresh spinach

6 eggs

2 tablespoons (28 ml) coconut milk or heavy cream

Per serving: 143 calories, 10 g fat, 10 g protein, 4 g carbohydrate, 2 g dietary fiber, 2 g net carbs

Eggs with Vermouth

The slightly bitter, herbal tang of vermouth makes these eggs very sophisticated. I served mine with a side of thick-cut peppered bacon. What could be bad?

Put your medium-sized skillet over medium heat. When it's hot, melt the butter and crack in the eggs. Let them cook for a minute or so and then add the vermouth and cover the skillet. Let the eggs cook for 2 to 3 minutes and then check. (You want the whites to be set, but the yolks still runny. Give the eggs another minute if they need it.) Plate and top with the parsley.

1 tablespoon (14 g) butter

3 eggs

1 tablespoon (15 ml) dry vermouth

1½ teaspoons minced parsley

Per serving: 316 calories, 25 g fat, 17 g protein, 3 g carbohydrate, trace dietary fiber, 3 g net carbs

Chicken Salad Scramble

When faced with leftover chicken, I usually make chicken salad, but not on days when the temperature drops into the single digits. I decided to put those flavors into my breakfast eggs, and the result was wonderful.

In a medium-sized skillet over medium heat, sauté the celery and scallions in the fat or oil for just a couple of minutes. (You want them to retain their crunch.) Add the chicken to the skillet and let it warm through.

In the meanwhile, scramble the eggs with the mustard in a bowl. Pour into the skillet and scramble till set. Plate and serve immediately!

¼ cup (30 g) finely diced celery

2 scallions, sliced thin, including the crisp part of the green

1½ tablespoons (21 g) chicken fat, (25 ml) avocado oil, or (21 g) lard

⅓ cup (47 g) diced cooked chicken

3 eggs

1 teaspoon spicy brown mustard

Per serving: 552 calories, 44 g fat, 32 g protein, 5 g carbohydrate, 1 g dietary fiber, 4 g net carbs

Chipotle Poached Eggs

Years ago, I fell in love with eggs poached in Creole tomato sauce. I've been poaching eggs in various sauces ever since. Note that this uses chipotle salsa, the kind usually served with chips, not the chipotle hot sauce in the shaker bottle.

Put your 8-inch (20 cm) nonstick skillet over medium heat. Add the salsa, water, and beef fat or bacon grease, let it warm, and stir together. Spread the mixture across the bottom of the skillet.

Carefully crack in the eggs. Turn the burner to low, cover the skillet, and let the eggs poach until done to your liking. That's it!

SERVES
1

¼ cup (65 g) chipotle salsa

1 tablespoon (15 ml) water

1 teaspoon beef fat or bacon grease

3 eggs

Per serving: 253 calories, 18 g fat, 17 g protein, 6 g carbohydrate, 1 g dietary fiber, 5 g net carbs

Pepper Poached Eggs

This recipe happened because Keith the Organic Gardening God bestowed a harvest of fresh paprika peppers upon me. These are about the size of jalapeños, but sweet, red, and only very mildly spicy. If you can't get paprika peppers, pick something with those qualities.

Put a smallish heavy skillet over medium heat and melt the coconut oil. Throw in the veggies. Let the pepper and onion sauté until they've softened. Add the coconut milk and stir everything up. Bring the mixture it to a simmer and let it cook for just a minute or two. Season it with salt and pepper. Now break the eggs into the skillet, cover the skillet, and turn the heat to medium-low. Let the eggs poach, checking often, until done to your liking. Plate, scrape any lingering sauce over the eggs, and serve immediately.

SERVES
1

1 tablespoon (14 g) coconut oil

2 tablespoons (11 g) minced fresh paprika pepper

2 tablespoons (20 g) minced onion

¼ cup (60 ml) coconut milk

Salt and ground black pepper, to taste

3 eggs

Per serving: 436 calories, 39 g fat, 18 g protein, 6 g carbohydrate, 1 g dietary fiber, 5 g net carbs

Eggs with Peas and Mint

SERVES 2

This unusual combination is easy, quick, great tasting, and very filling. Yes, peas are a legume, but because they're edible raw, I consider them Paleo-friendly.

Steam the peas until tender. (My frozen ones took 10 minutes in the microwave.) Drain the peas.

Place a medium-sized skillet over medium-low heat. When the skillet is hot, add the eggs, peas, and mint. Scramble slowly till set. Pour the butter on top. Plate and serve immediately!

½ cup (75 g) fresh or (65 g) frozen green peas

4 eggs, scrambled

1 tablespoon (6 g) fresh mint leaves, minced

1 tablespoon (14 g) butter or other fat, melted

Per serving: 213 calories, 15 g fat, 13 g protein, 7 g carbohydrate, 2 g dietary fiber, 5 g net carbs

> ## note
> I used frozen peas because it was January, with no fresh ones to be found, but if you have fresh peas, use 'em!

Sausage Hash with Eggs

SERVES 3

I was torn as to whether this went in the pork chapter or the egg chapter. Either way, it's filling and delicious, and it's great any time of day.

Put a big, heavy skillet over medium heat and brown and crumble the Breakfast Sausage.

When some fat has cooked out of the sausage, add the onion and pepper. (Feel free to add a dollop of bacon grease if needed.) Stir it up and then spread it in a layer in the pan. Keep cooking, stirring, and turning it all over every 3 to 4 minutes until the veggies are soft and the sausage has some brown flecks.

Spread the hash evenly in the skillet and break the eggs over it. Cover the skillet, turn down the burner a little, and keep cooking until the whites are set and the yolks are done to your liking.

⅓ of the recipe for Breakfast Sausage, (1 pound [455 g]) (See page 108.)

½ of a medium onion, diced

½ of a medium green pepper, diced

Bacon grease (optional)

6 eggs

Per serving: 539 calories, 43 g fat, 30 g protein, 7 g carbohydrate, 1 g dietary fiber, 6 g net carbs

The World's Most Nutritious Breakfast

There is no diet that wouldn't be nutritionally enhanced by eating this once or twice a week. It's super tasty and filling, too.

If you don't have a bacon grease jar, you'll want to cook the bacon first. But why don't you have a bacon grease jar?! Anyway, see to it your bacon is crisp.

Remove the bacon to a paper towel–lined plate. Throw in the onion and tomato and let them sauté, stirring occasionally.

Meanwhile, snip the chicken livers into bite-sized bits. (Kitchen shears are good for this.) Break and scramble the eggs into a bowl.

When the onion is soft and translucent, turning golden, and the tomato has melted down a bit, throw in the liver. Sauté, stirring often, until the outsides have changed color and the juices have stopped running red, but no more! (Overcooked liver is a culinary tragedy.) Pour in the eggs and scramble till set.

Plate, crumble the bacon over it, and serve immediately.

2 slices of bacon

1 tablespoon (14 g) bacon grease

½ of a small onion, diced fine

½ of a medium tomato, diced

2 chicken livers

3 eggs

Per serving: 502 calories, 35 g fat, 33 g protein, 11 g carbohydrate, 2 g dietary fiber, 9 g net carbs

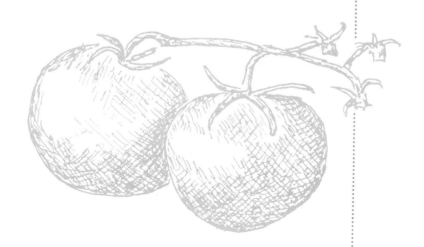

Poultry

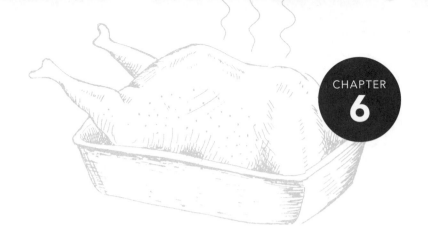

Somehow America has become fixated on boneless, skinless chicken breast. I blame it on Low-Fat Mania, but I do not understand it. To me, the boneless, skinless breast is the blandest and most boring form chicken could possibly take. Its only virtue is that it cooks quickly.

Further, boneless, skinless breast is not a whole food. Skin is full of gelatin, excellent for joints, hair, nails, and gut health. Bones are the source of bone broth, one of the most magical ingredients in your kitchen. With a whole chicken, you get giblets, sneaking a few organ meats into your diet. That is way more Paleo. We will be using boneless, skinless chicken in this chapter, but only when it's essential to the dish.

Some people are squicked out by chicken with bones and skin; it reminds them that they're eating an animal, something that lived and breathed. I hope you don't feel this way, but if you do, you need to reach deep and find your inner hunter.

So let's start with the whole chicken, that coveted Sunday dinner special of years gone by. This is, after all, the chicken our ancestors knew.

Savory Roast Chicken

Whole chickens take an hour or so to roast, but they are super easy, often inexpensive, and let diners choose white or dark meat as they like. Plus you'll have a carcass to make broth from!

Preheat the oven to 375°F (190°C or gas mark 5).

First, remove the giblets from the body cavity. Put all but the liver in a small saucepan, cover with water, and set on a low burner. Simmer till they're tender.

Wash the chicken and pat it dry with paper towels.

In a small dish, mix together the oil with the Creole Seasoning and hot sauce.

Using clean hands, loosen the skin on the chicken as much as you can, while leaving it intact. Spoon the seasoned oil under the skin and use your hands to massage it around to coat as much of the chicken's meat as possible. Use about half the oil this way, getting it under as much of the skin as you can. Rub some of the seasoned oil on the outside of the skin, too. If there's any left, spoon it into the cavity.

If you want the chicken to look tidy, tie the ends of the drumsticks together with cotton string or thread.

Place the chicken on a rack in a roasting pan and slide 'er into the oven. Roast for about 1 hour or until a meat thermometer stuck in the thickest part of the thigh registers 165°F (74°C). Wiggle the drumsticks. If they move easily, that sucker is done.

Remove the chicken from the oven and let it sit for 15 to 20 minutes for the juices to settle back into the meat before you carve it.

What about those giblets? When the heart and gizzard are tender, drop the liver into the water, turn off the burner, and cover the pot. The retained heat will cook the liver. You can use these in gravy or make Totally Inauthentic Dirty "Rice" (see page 137).

SERVES 5

1 whole chicken
(4 pounds or 1.8 kg)

¼ cup (60 ml) olive oil

2 tablespoons (30 g) Creole Seasoning (See page 35.)

1 tablespoon (14 ml) Frank's Hot Sauce

Per serving: 763 calories, 63 g fat, 45 g protein, 3 g carbohydrate, 1 g dietary fiber, 2 g net carbs

note

Some of the olive oil—and, of course, some of the chicken fat—will cook out, so that calorie count above is higher than it actually will be. That fat will be fabulous for cooking, by the way. Pour it off the drippings and save it!

Chicken Nuggets

Or, if you prefer, you can make tenders. Just cut 'em in strips instead of squares. Crunchy on the outside, moist on the inside, these are sure to please the whole family. This one does call for boneless, skinless chicken.

Preheat the oven to its lowest temperature.

Cut the chicken into chunks. (Mine were about 1½ inches × 2 inches [3.8 × 5 cm], but it's up to you. The smaller the bits, the more coating you'll use, but the quicker they'll cook.)

Run the pork rinds through your food processor till they're crumbs, add the Creole Seasoning, and pulse to mix. Dump this into a pie plate.

In another pie plate, beat the eggs with the water till they're well blended.

Put a big heavy skillet over medium heat and add some fat. You want it to be about ½ inch (1.3 cm) deep, and, should you have a thermometer, you're shooting for 375°F (190°C). (I bought one of the new induction burners largely because it lets me hold a specific temperature. It's very helpful.)

Okay, make an assembly line: chicken chunks, egg wash, pork rind crumbs, and a plate on the end for the coated nuggets. Use a fork to dip each nugget in the egg wash and then the crumbs, coating each completely. Add the nuggets to fill your skillet without crowding it. (You want about 1 inch [2.5 cm] between nuggets.) Fry them for 3 to 4 minutes. Go start breading the next batch.

When the timer beeps, flip the frying nuggets and reset the timer for another 3 to 4 minutes. Go bread more nuggets! As each batch is done, transfer them to a shallow baking sheet in the oven to keep warm—or just serve them in batches, which is what I did. Add more lard to the skillet as it is needed to maintain that ½- inch (1.3 cm) depth and keep frying nuggets till they're all done.

2 pounds (910 g) boneless, skinless chicken breasts or thighs

7 ounces (200 g) pork rinds (two big bags)

2 tablespoons (22 g) Creole Seasoning (See page 35.)

4 eggs

2 tablespoons (28 ml) water

Lard or other fat

Per serving: 231 calories, 7 g fat, 38 g protein, 2 g carbohydrate, trace dietary fiber, 2 g net carbs

note

Serve these nuggets with the dipping sauce of your choice. Try the Honey Mustard Dressing and Dipping Sauce on page 33.

Pesto Chicken Pouches

This dish features chicken and vegetables, all together, and not a single pan to wash. How great is that? Tester Rebecca called this "wonderfully easy, and very, very tasty." She also suggested trying it with other vegetables. You can serve these over a bed of Caulirice (see page 128) or Zoodles, which is zucchini that is cut with a spiral cutter and lightly cooked. Pile the chicken and veggies on it, pouring all the liquid from the foil over it, too.

Preheat the oven to 450°F (230°C or gas mark 8).

Start with a little prep: Snap the ends off the asparagus where they naturally want to break. Cut them in 2-inch (5 cm) lengths. Cut the tomato into 8 slices.

In a small bowl, mix together the pesto and mayo.

Tear four sheets of foil big enough to completely wrap a serving of the chicken and vegetables. Put a sheet of foil on the counter. Put a breast or thigh (or possibly 2 thighs, if they're kinda puny) in the center of the foil. Season the chicken to taste with salt and pepper. Spread 2 tablespoons (31 g) of the sauce over the chicken. Lay a couple of slices of tomato on top, and arrange the asparagus around it.

Fold the foil over, rolling down the edge, and then roll in the ends. Repeat until you have four packets and no more ingredients. Lay the packets in your roasting pan, just in case there is a leak. Bake the packets for 25 to 30 minutes. Serve right from the foil.

1 pound (455 g) asparagus

1 big tomato, or 2 little ones

¼ cup (65 g) pesto sauce

¼ cup (60 g) Good Ol' Mayonnaise (See page 30.)

24 ounces (680 g) boneless, skinless chicken thighs or breasts

Salt

Ground black pepper

Per serving: 459 calories, 38 g fat, 25 g protein, 5 g carbohydrate, 2 g dietary fiber, 3 g net carbs

note

If it's summer and you hate the idea of a 450°F (230°C or gas mark 8) oven in your kitchen, you can grill these.

Pesto-Nut Chicken

SERVES
6

Asked "Would you make this again?" tester Hanftka replied, "Yes, in fact I have already made it again!"

Preheat the oven to 350°F (180°C or gas mark 4).

Spread the pecans in a shallow baking sheet, and put them in the oven, while it heats, for 6 minutes.

Place the chicken in a roasting pan and coat with the pesto.

When the oven timer beeps, pull out the pecans and turn the oven up to 375°F (190°C or gas mark 5).

Dump the pecans in a food processor. Pulse until they're chopped to a medium consistency. Spread them on a rimmed plate.

Roll the pesto-coated chicken in the pecans, making a nice thick coating. Put the chicken back in the roasting pan, skin side up. Roast for 50 to 60 minutes or until the juices run clear.

¾ cup (75 g) pecans

3 pounds (1.4 kg) chicken (Use thighs, breasts, or both, with skin, as you choose.)

¾ cup (195 g) pesto sauce

Per serving: 576 calories, 46 g fat, 35 g protein, 5 g carbohydrate, 1 g dietary fiber, 4 g net carbs

Simply Saucy Chicken

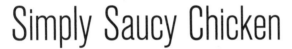

SERVES
6

Tester Rebecca calls this "so delicious, and so easy to make." She adds, "I will absolutely keep making it over and over again as long as I live." Serve it on a bed of Caulirice (see page 128).

Preheat the oven to 350°F (180°C or gas mark 4).

Lay the chicken in a roasting pan. (I'd use a glass pan, such as Pyrex, for this because it's nonreactive.)

In a bowl, mix together everything else and pour it over the chicken. Bake the chicken for 40 minutes. If the sauce is a bit watery, which can happen if the chicken is very juicy, pour it into a nonreactive saucepan and give it few minutes of simmering on the stove. Serve the sauce over the chicken.

2½ pounds (1 kg) chicken (Use breasts, thighs, or both.)

1 jar (16 ounces, or 455 g) salsa

36 drops of English toffee–flavored liquid stevia extract

1½ teaspoons honey

2 tablespoons (30 g) spicy brown mustard

Per serving: 236 calories, 6 g fat, 37 g protein, 7 g carbohydrate, 1 g dietary fiber, 6 g net carbs

Chicken and Bok Choy Stir-Fry

This is fast, simple, and good. What more could you ask from a meal? Oh, yeah, it's nutritious and cheap, too. You can serve this over Caulirice (see page 128) if you like, but we ate it as is. This is just one of 100 great dinners you can put together in a flash if you keep stir-fry sauces in your fridge.

Slice the chicken into thin strips. (This is easier if it's half frozen.)

How you cut the bok choy will depend on how big it is. I had a 1-pound (455 g) head, so I broke off about half of it and cut it crosswise at ½-inch (1.3 cm) intervals. If you're lucky enough to find little baby heads of bok choy, quarter them lengthwise and use them that way. Either way, use both the leaves and the stems.

Halve the onion lengthwise, rather than through the equator. Peel it and slice it lengthwise, into about ¼-inch (6 mm) thick slices.

Measure the stir-fry sauce and have it by the stove.

It's cooking time! Put a wok or big skillet over the highest heat. Melt half of the lard or oil and let it get good and hot. Throw in the chicken and stir-fry till all the pink is gone. Scoop it out and reserve on a plate.

Melt the rest of the lard or oil. When it's hot, add the bok choy and onion. Stir fry for about 3 minutes until the onion is just getting tender-crisp.

Return the chicken to the skillet, add the stir-fry sauce, and stir it all up. Let it simmer for a couple of minutes and then serve immediately.

12 ounces (340 g) boneless, skinless chicken breasts or thighs

8 ounces (225 g) bok choy

1 medium onion

¼ cup (60 ml) Basic Stir-Fry Sauce (See page 33.)

3 tablespoons (42 g) lard or coconut oil, divided

Per serving: 296 calories, 16 g fat, 27 g protein, 8 g carbohydrate, 1 g dietary fiber, 7 g net carbs

Lemon Tarragon Chicken

SERVES
4

This recipe is chicken in a creamy lemon-tarragon sauce, with an elegance that belies the ease with which it's made. Try nestling the chicken into a bed of Caulirice (see page 128) and pouring the sauce over the whole thing. Wow.

Preheat the oven to 400°F (200°C or gas mark 6).

Season the chicken with salt and pepper all over, lay it in a stove-top-safe roasting pan—8 × 8-inches (20.3 × 20.3 cm) is about right for four thighs—and roast it for 30 minutes. (Because you'll be putting the pan over a burner later, don't use a glass baking dish such as Pyrex; it's not stove-top safe.)

When the timer beeps, baste the chicken with the grease collecting in the pan. Now let it roast till done, for another 15 to 20 minutes.

While the chicken is roasting, grate the zest of the lemon and squeeze every drop of juice out of it that you can.

Pull the pan out of the oven and remove the chicken to a plate somewhere warm. Pour all but 1 to 2 tablespoons (15 to 28 ml) of the grease out of the pan, but retain the nice brown drippings. Put the pan on a stove burner over low heat. Add the lemon juice, tarragon, and coconut milk. Use a spatula to stir, scraping all the brown stuff off the bottom of the pan into the sauce. Use the edge of the spatula to break up any lumps of brown stuff to better dissolve the flavor into the sauce.

Bring the sauce to a simmer and let it cook for 5 minutes, to thicken just a bit. Stir in the lemon zest and then serve the sauce spooned over the chicken.

24 ounces (683 g) chicken thighs (4 pieces)

Salt

Ground black pepper

½ lemon

1 tablespoon (4 g) fresh tarragon, minced

1 cup (235 ml) coconut milk

Per serving: 390 calories, 32 g fat, 23 g protein, 4 g carbohydrate, 1 g dietary fiber, 3 g net carbs

Chicken with Artichokes and Olives

It's Mediterranean goodness that's quick and easy enough for a weeknight. Serve with Caulirice (see page 128) or Zoodles (see recipe intro on page 67). You can use fresh artichokes if you like, but extracting 14 ounces (390 g) worth of hearts is a lot of work.

Strip the skin off the chicken. (You can buy them skinless if you like, but they'll be more expensive, and you'll miss the opportunity to make Chicken Chips on page 46.) Pour 2 tablespoons (28 ml) of the oil from the olives into your big, heavy skillet, put it over medium heat, and add the thighs, boney side up. Start them browning a bit.

In the meanwhile, chop the olives. (If they're not pitted to start with, the easiest way is to squish each one with your thumb. The pits will then flick out easily. But if you can find pitted olives in olive oil, go for it.)

Turn the chicken! Start it browning on the bottom.

In a small bowl, stir the garlic into the lemon juice and water, along with the pepper.

Okay, the chicken is golden on both sides. Arrange the chopped olives and artichoke hearts around and over the thighs and pour in the lemon juice/garlic mixture. Cover the skillet with a tilted lid, leaving a crack for steam to escape, turn the burner to a low simmer, and let the whole thing cook for 25 to 30 minutes.

When the chicken is done, remove it to a platter. Turn up the burner and boil the sauce down a little more, till it gets syrupy. Add salt to taste, if needed.

Serve the chicken with the sauce, olives, and artichokes spooned over it.

6 chicken thighs

24 olives, packed in olive oil

5 cloves of garlic, crushed

¼ cup (60 ml) lemon juice

¼ cup (60 ml) water

½ teaspoon ground black pepper

14 ounces (390 g) quartered artichoke hearts, frozen if you can find 'em, otherwise canned

Salt (optional)

Per serving: 258 calories, 16 g fat, 19 g protein, 10 g carbohydrate, 4 g dietary fiber, 6 g net carbs

Roast Chicken with Creamy Sun-Dried Tomato Sauce

This is so easy it's ridiculous, and yet it's so delicious your family will get confused and start looking around for company. Serve this with a bed of Caulirice (see page 128) to soak up the sauce.

Preheat the oven to 400°F (200°C or gas mark 6).

Season the chicken with salt and pepper all over and arrange it in a metal baking pan. (Metal browns better than glass, plus you need to cook this on the stove later, too.) Roast the chicken till it's done. (Mine took about 1 hour, but then, I had some hellaciously big thighs.) You want it done enough that the juices run clear and the drippings in the pan are turning brown and crunchy.

Remove the pan from the oven and transfer the chicken to a platter. Pour the excess grease off the drippings and put the pan over a low burner.

Crush in the garlic and stir it around for just a minute. Now add the tomatoes and coconut milk. Stir the mixture with a spatula, scraping up all the nice brown stuff, dissolving it into the sauce.

Let the sauce simmer a few minutes till it thickens up a bit and then serve the sauce spooned over the chicken.

2 pounds (900 g) chicken pieces (Thighs are good for this, but use what you like.)

Salt

Ground black pepper

1 clove of garlic

⅓ cup (18 g) chopped sun-dried tomatoes

1 cup (235 ml) coconut milk or heavy cream

Per serving: 457 calories, 35 g fat, 31 g protein, 4 g carbohydrate, 1 g dietary fiber, 3 g net carbs

Rosemary Chicken and Radishes

SERVES
4

Keith the Organic Gardening God—my next door neighbor— showed up with a huge bunch of fresh rosemary, inspiring this recipe. As for the roasted radishes? They're astonishing.

Preheat the oven to 375°F (190°C or gas mark 5).

Season the chicken with salt and pepper all over and arrange it in a dark, heavy, metal baking pan.

Trim the radishes if they need it and then whack 'em each in half. Arrange the radishes flat sides down around the chicken.

In a bowl, mix together the oil, rosemary, and garlic and spoon it over the chicken and radishes. Roast the chicken for 30 minutes and then baste it well with the combined oil and grease. Baste the radishes, too. Roast the chicken for another 20 minutes and then check to see if the chicken is brown and crisp. If not, give it another 10 minutes or so.

Serve the chicken and the radishes with some of the pan juices spooned over them.

4 chicken thighs

Salt

Ground black pepper

¼ cup (60 ml) olive oil

1 tablespoon (2 g) minced fresh rosemary

1 clove of garlic, crushed

50 or so radishes

Per serving: 330 calories, 28 g fat, 17 g protein, 2 g carbohydrate, 1 g dietary fiber, 1 g net carbs

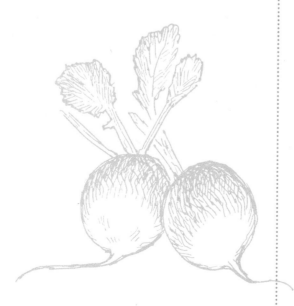

Dana's Failed Fricassee Triumph

I tried doing a Paleo riff on a chicken fricassee recipe I'd seen. It was tasty, but unpleasantly greasy. So I turned it into roast chicken with a quick pan sauce and wow!

Preheat the oven to 400°F (200°C or gas mark 6).

Season the chicken with salt and pepper all over and lay it in a metal roasting pan. Throw the chicken in the oven and roast it for 30 minutes.

When the timer beeps, baste the chicken with the fat that will have accumulated in the bottom of the pan. At the same time, assess your chicken for signs of doneness. (The timing will depend some on the size of the chicken thighs.) They'll probably need at least another 15 minutes. You want the skin crisp and golden, the juices running clear, and—this is important—the goopy drippings to have turned gloriously brown and crunchy in the bottom of the roasting pan. When you see this, pull the roasting pan out of the oven and remove the chicken to a platter. Pour off all but a couple of teaspoons of fat. Put the pan on a burner over medium-low heat.

Add the garlic and sauté it in the chicken grease for a minute or so. Now add everything else and whisk it together, scraping up and dissolving all that crunchy brown stuff. Bring this sauce to a simmer. Let the sauce cook for 5 minutes or so till it reduces enough to become slightly syrupy. Serve the sauce over the chicken.

SERVES 4

4 chicken thighs

Salt

Ground black pepper

4 cloves of garlic, crushed

1 tablespoon (4 g) poultry seasoning

1 cup (235 ml) chicken broth

2 tablespoons (32 g) tomato paste

Per serving: 222 calories, 15 g fat, 18 g protein, 3 g carbohydrate, trace dietary fiber, 3 g net carbs

The-Last-of-the-Thanksgiving-Leftovers Hash

SERVES 3

A full week after Thanksgiving, I came up with this recipe to use up enough of the remaining turkey that I could break down the carcass for soup. Enough is enough. Turns out, this is really great!

Dice the sweet potato into ¼-inch (6 mm) cubes. Put a big, heavy skillet over medium heat, melt 2 tablespoons (28 g) of the bacon grease, and throw in the sweet potato. Spread it into an even layer, cover the skillet, and let it cook.

In the meanwhile, dice the onion and mushrooms to about the same size as the sweet potato. Stir the onion and mushrooms into the sweet potato, adding another 1 tablespoon (14 g) of grease, spread it into an even layer again, and re-cover the skillet.

Check on the veggies—is the sweet potato beginning to soften? The onion, too? Okay, stir in the turkey, with the last of the bacon grease. Spread it out, re-cover the pan, and let it cook for 5 minutes. Repeat the process, making sure to scrape up any nice brown stuff from the bottom of the skillet as you turn it all over.

When the veggies are soft and the turkey is hot through, stir in the gravy, should you be lucky enough to have some. (I always make vats of the stuff.) Season the dish with salt and pepper to taste. Let the whole thing cook for another 5 minutes and then dish it up.

1 medium sweet potato

¼ cup (55 g) bacon grease or leftover turkey grease if you have any, divided

1 medium onion

4 ounces (115 g) mushrooms

2 cups (280 g) diced turkey

¼ cup (60 g) gravy, homemade if you have it (optional)

Salt

Ground black pepper

Per serving: 403 calories, 25 g fat, 24 g protein, 20 g carbohydrate, 3 g dietary fiber, 17 g net carbs

Fish and Seafood

It is my considered opinion that fish come in a range of Paleo-ness, depending on how big they are and how far out to sea they live. People without power cruisers probably weren't getting as many big tuna and swordfish as they were clams and mussels, which can be gathered by the shore.

At spawning time, salmon could simply be speared, as could fish in local ponds and streams.

Still, the vast majority of fish fall into the "edible raw" category, although only when strictly fresh, of course. For these recipes, I worked with what wild-caught fish I could find at local grocery stores and at Costco. If you have a fisherman or woman in the family, so much the better! Try some of these preparations with whatever can be caught locally.

Glazed Salmon

Have you noticed how many of my recipes involve a skillet? That's because it's the quickest way to cook so many things, and it's so often the most satisfactory. Here, you'll turn out salmon fit for company in 10 minutes.

In a big, heavy skillet over medium-high heat, start searing the salmon in 2 tablespoons (28 ml) of the oil.

In the meanwhile, stir together the wine, mustard, and stevia in a bowl.

When the salmon has a little color on both sides, remove it to a plate, but keep it by the stove. Add the rest of the oil and the shallot to the skillet. Sauté, stirring frequently, for just a couple of minutes. Pour in the wine mixture and stir it all around, scraping up all the flavorsome stuff on the bottom of the pan. Let it simmer for a few minutes till it cooks down about halfway.

Put the salmon back in the skillet, flipping it once to coat both sides. Let it cook for another couple of minutes till you're sure it's done through. (I watch for the red line in the center to fade to pink.)

Plate the salmon, scrape the rest of the pan liquid over the fish, dividing it equally, and serve immediately.

1 salmon fillet (24 ounces, or 680 g), cut into 4 servings

¼ cup (60 ml) avocado oil or other fat, divided

¼ cup (60 ml) dry white wine

1 tablespoon (15 g) plus 1 teaspoon whole grain Dijon mustard

24 drops of English toffee–flavored liquid stevia extract

¼ cup (40 g) minced shallots

Per serving: 339 calories, 20 g fat, 34 g protein, 2 g carbohydrate, trace dietary fiber, 2 g net carbs

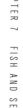

CHAPTER 7 FISH AND SEAFOOD

Mustard Salmon

This is fast and easy, and my husband said it might be the best salmon I ever made. Of course, he is remarkably fond of salmon.

Preheat the oven to 350°F (180°C or gas mark 4). Line a baking sheet with non-stick foil.

Season the salmon lightly with salt and pepper and then spread each non-skin-side with ½ tablespoon of the mustard. Lay it skin-side down on the foil. Repeat with the other three fillets.

Bake the salmon for about 15 minutes.

In the meanwhile, over medium-low heat, melt the butter in a skillet and add the crumbs. Cook the crumbs, stirring often, until they brown a little and become very crisp.

When the salmon is done, plate it, and spread ¼ of the crumb mixture over each fillet. Serve the salmon immediately.

SERVES 4

1 salmon fillet (24 ounces, or 680 g), cut into 4 servings

Salt

Ground black pepper

2 tablespoons (30 g) spicy brown mustard

1½ teaspoons butter or other fat

½ cup (50 g) Italian-Seasoned Pork Rind Crumbs (See page 37.)

Per serving: 286 calories, 12 g fat, 42 g protein, 1 g carbohydrate, trace dietary fiber, 1 g net carbs

Slammin' Salmon Stacks

The Mega Food Stacks on page 93 were such a success, I thought I'd try expanding on the concept with salmon.

In a big skillet over medium heat fry the bacon until crisp. Remove the bacon to a plate and reserve. Pour half of the grease into a second skillet and put both skillets over medium heat.

Sprinkle the meat side of the salmon fillets liberally with the Creole Seasoning and lay them skin-side down in the first skillet.

When the salmon is halfway done—look at the edges to check for the color change—flip it. Now crack the eggs into the other skillet and cover it. Fry the eggs till the whites are done, but the yolks are still runny.

Put each fillet on a plate. Spread 2 ounces (55 g) of guacamole on each. Now layer two slices of bacon—snap 'em in half to make them fit—over that, top each with a fried egg, and serve immediately.

SERVES 4

8 slices of bacon

1 salmon fillet (24 ounces, or 680 g), cut into 4 servings

Creole Seasoning (See page 35.)

4 eggs

8 ounces (225 g) guacamole, divided

Per serving: 424 calories, 25 g fat, 44 g protein, 5 g carbohydrate, 1 g dietary fiber, 4 g net carbs

Salmon with Shallots and Capers

Here's an eclectic mix of flavors that turn out delicious.

Use the least-sticky skillet you have that will fit your salmon. Give it a shot of coconut oil spray if you have it and put it over medium heat.

In the meanwhile, season the salmon with salt and pepper on both sides.

When the skillet is hot, add 1 tablespoon (15 ml) of the oil and slosh it around to cover the bottom of the pan. Add the salmon, skin side down, and cook it for 3 to 4 minutes. Flip the salmon and give it another 3 to 4 minutes. Remove it to a plate and keep it warm.

Add the rest of the oil to the skillet and throw in the shallot. Stir it around, sautéing for just a minute or so. Now add the salsa, vinegar, and capers and stir it up, scraping up the tasty brown stuff from the bottom of the skillet. Turn up the heat a little and let this mixture boil hard for a couple of minutes to thicken.

Put the salmon back in the skillet, cover it, and let it cook for another minute or two. (The timing will depend on how thick your fillets are.) When the salmon is flaky, plate it and spoon the sauce over the top to serve.

SERVES 4

1 salmon fillet (24 ounces, or 680 g), cut into 4 servings

Salt

Ground black pepper

2 tablespoons (28 ml) olive oil, divided

1 shallot, sliced paper-thin

¼ cup (65 g) chunky salsa

2 tablespoons (28 ml) red wine vinegar

1 tablespoon (9 g) capers, drained and chopped

Per serving: 265 calories, 13 g fat, 34 g protein, 2 g carbohydrate, trace dietary fiber, 2 g net carbs

note

A little parsley would be nice in this, should you feel like snipping some.

Sea Bass with Bacon Vinaigrette

Can't find sea bass? You can substitute cod or halibut, and it will work just fine.

Let's deal with the bacon first. Put a big skillet over medium-low heat and start it cooking. You'll want it crisp.

Season the bass with salt and pepper. When the bacon is crisp, remove it from the pan and reserve on a plate. Pour off all but 2 tablespoons (28 ml) of the grease. Throw in the fish. Cook it for about 5 minutes per side or until flaky. (The timing will depend on the thickness of your filets.)

When the fish is done, plate it and keep it somewhere warm.

Pour the dressing into the skillet and stir it around, scraping up any brown bits and mixing the grease with the dressing. Pour this over the fish, top each serving with 2 slices of bacon, and serve immediately.

SERVES 3

6 slices of bacon

1 bass fillet (1 pound, or 455 g), cut into 3 servings

Salt and ground black pepper, to taste

⅓ cup (80 ml) Apple-y Dressing (See page 32.)

Per serving: 472 calories, 37 g fat, 33 g protein, 1 g carbohydrate, trace dietary fiber, 1 g net carbs

Pepper-Lime Snapper

This recipe has everything you could want. It's super-simple, lightning quick, and utterly delicious. That Nice Boy I Married went on and on about this.

Put your skillet, preferably nonstick, over medium-low heat. While it's warming, season both sides of the snapper with salt and then liberally with pepper—not just a light sprinkling.

When the skillet is hot, add the oil. Throw in the fish, skin side down. Cook the fish for about 3 minutes. Flip, and cook it for another 3 minutes, until the fish is flaky clear through.

Squeeze the lime evenly over the fish, sprinkle the fish with a little extra pepper, and serve immediately.

SERVES 4

1 whole red snapper (1 pound, or 455 g), cut into 4 servings

Salt and ground black pepper, to taste

2 tablespoons (28 ml) avocado oil

½ of a lime

Per serving: 176 calories, 8 g fat, 23 g protein, 1 g carbohydrate, trace dietary fiber, 1 g net carbs

Trout with Tomatoes, Scallions, and Capers

This dish is simple and delicious—especially if you can get fresh-caught trout.

Preheat the oven to 350°F (180°C or gas mark 4).

In the meanwhile, lay Mr. Trout in a pan. (I used a glass Pyrex dish.) Pour the oil over the top. Rub it all over, including inside, and then season the fish with salt and pepper inside and out.

Scatter the tomato, scallions, and capers evenly over the trout, covering it. (It's okay if some falls along the sides, too.) Bake, uncovered, for 30 minutes and then serve immediately.

1 whole rainbow trout, cleaned

1 tablespoon (15 ml) olive oil

Salt and ground black pepper, to taste

1 medium tomato, diced

2 scallions, sliced

2 tablespoons (17 g) capers, drained and chopped

Per serving: 393 calories, 21 g fat, 43 g protein, 8 g carbohydrate, 2 g dietary fiber, 6 g net carbs

Blackened Red Snapper

Warning: Cooking hot peppers at high temperature creates vapors that will make you cough. Turn on the vent fan, open a window, or do whatever you need to do.

In a small bowl, mix all of the seasonings together.

Lay the snapper, skin-side up, on your cutting board. Use a thin, sharp bladed knife to make 3 or 4 shallow cuts across the skin of each fillet. (This keeps the fish from curling up as it cooks.)

Flip the fish and sprinkle the meaty side of the fish liberally with the spice mixture. If you've got the time, let this sit for 30 minutes to 1 hour.

Put a big, heavy skillet over medium-high heat. When it's hot, melt the lard. Throw in the fish, seasoned side down. Let the fish cook for 3 minutes or until it is well browned. Flip and cook the other side for 2 to 3 minutes. Plate the fish and serve immediately.

1½ tablespoons (17 g) Creole Seasoning (See page 35.)

1 teaspoon erythritol

1 teaspoon ground black pepper

1 pinch of cayenne pepper, or to taste

1 red snapper fillet (24 ounces, or 680 g), cut into 6 servings

1 tablespoon (14 g) lard

Per serving: 137 calories, 4 g fat, 24 g protein, 1 g carbohydrate, trace dietary fiber, 1 g net carbs

Cod with Spicy Lemon-Tomato Sauce and Pine Nuts

SERVES
4

I used Rao's brand of arrabiata sauce, which has no sugar, bad oils, or other junk added. Look for it.

First, put a big skillet (I like ceramic nonstick for this) over medium low heat and add the pine nuts. Stir the nuts until they're lightly golden and then remove them to a plate and reserve. Increase the heat to medium. Season the cod with salt and pepper on both sides.

Add the oil or lard to the skillet, slosh it around, and then add the fish. Let it sear for a minute or two, flip, and sear the other side.

In the meanwhile, mix the arrabiata sauce and the lemon juice together in a small bowl. Pour this mixture evenly over the cod and cover the skillet with a tilted lid—in other words, leave a crack open for steam to escape. Let the fish cook for 5 to 7 minutes or till it is flaky. (The timing will depend some on how thick your fish is.)

Plate the cod, spooning the remaining sauce from the skillet over each fillet. Top each with 1 tablespoon (9 g) of pine nuts and serve immediately.

¼ cup (35 g) pine nuts

1 cod fillet (24 ounces, or 680 g)

Salt and ground black pepper, to taste

¼ cup (60 ml) olive oil or (55 g) lard

1 cup (245 g) arrabiata pasta sauce

½ cup (120 ml) lemon juice

Per serving: 235 calories, 10 g fat, 32 g protein, 4 g carbohydrate, 1 g dietary fiber, 3 g net carbs

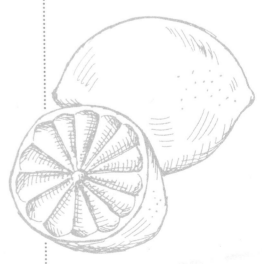

Simple Spiced Shrimp

SERVES
4

Simple is good! This recipe doubles or triples easily, too, though I wouldn't double or triple the oil.

Put a big, heavy skillet over medium-low heat and add the oil. Slosh it around to coat the bottom of the skillet and add the shrimp in a single layer. Let it cook for 3 or 4 minutes while you assemble your spices.

Flip the shrimp and sprinkle the spices over them. Let the shrimp cook for another 3 or 4 minutes, stir for a moment to make sure they're well-coated with the spices, and serve with plenty of napkins.

3 tablespoons (45 ml) olive oil

1 pound (455 g) easy-peel shrimp

2 cloves of garlic, crushed

2 teaspoons paprika

2 teaspoons Italian Seasoning

¼ teaspoon cayenne or a shot of Frank's Hot Sauce

Per serving: 218 calories, 12 g fat, 23 g protein, 3 g carbohydrate, 1 g dietary fiber, 2 g net carbs

Chipotle Lime Shrimp

SERVES
4

This one is for all you Mexican food fans, and I know you are legion. You can simplify this by using only one or the other fat, but the combo does taste mighty good.

Put a big, heavy skillet over medium-low heat and add the oil and butter. When the butter melts, swirl them together to cover the bottom of the pan and add the shrimp in a single layer.

Okay, the shrimp are pink on one side. Flip 'em! Let 'em sit for another 3 minutes or so. When the shrimp are pink through, stir in the hot sauce, lime juice, and cumin. Dish 'em up, scatter the cilantro over 'em, and serve with plenty of napkins.

2 tablespoons (28 ml) olive oil

1 tablespoon (14 g) butter

1 pound (455 g) raw, peeled shrimp

3 tablespoons (28 ml) chipotle hot sauce

2 tablespoons (30 ml) lime juice

½ teaspoon ground cumin

2 tablespoons (2 g) minced cilantro

Per serving: 210 calories, 12 g fat, 23 g protein, 2 g carbohydrate, trace dietary fiber, 2 g net carbs

Shrimp with Sun-Dried Tomatoes

This has a sort of American-Asian Fusion thing going on. For a totally different take, swap out the sriracha for Frank's Hot Sauce and sub a smidge of pesto for the sesame oil.

How much easier could this be? Put a big skillet over medium-high heat. Melt the coconut oil and throw in the shrimp.

Chop up the sun-dried tomatoes. (You want 'em fairly small, maybe pea-sized or smaller.)

Stir the shrimp, making sure they all get turned over.

Chop the onion to about the same size as the tomatoes. Are the shrimp getting pink through? Add the tomatoes and onion and stir it up. Add the sriracha and the sesame oil, too, and stir again. Let it all cook for another minute or 2 and then serve. It's up to you whether this is finger food or needs forks.

SERVES 4

2 tablespoons (28 g) coconut oil

1 pound (455 g) raw, peeled shrimp

¼ cup (28 g) chopped sun-dried tomatoes jarred in olive oil

¼ cup (40 g) diced red onion

2 teaspoons sriracha

½ teaspoon dark sesame oil

Per serving: 197 calories, 9 g fat, 23 g protein, 4 g carbohydrate, 1 g dietary fiber, 3 g net carbs

Spicy Skillet Shrimp

That Nice Boy I Married had a few friends in for a meeting. I put a plate of these in their midst, along with a stack of napkins, and got out of the way!

Put a big skillet (I really did use a bigger skillet than my standard cast-iron job for this) over medium-high heat and sauté the shrimp in the oil.

While the shrimp are cooking, stir together the lime juice, sriracha, and garlic in a bowl. When the shrimp are looking done through, pour the lime juice mixture over them and stir till they're all well coated. That's it!

SERVES 4

1 pound (455 g) raw, shelled shrimp, with tails

2 tablespoons (28 g) coconut oil

2 tablespoons (28 ml) lime juice

1 tablespoon (15 ml) sriracha, or to taste

2 cloves of garlic, crushed

Per serving: 184 calories, 9 g fat, 23 g protein, 2 g carbohydrate, trace dietary fiber, 2 g net carbs

Shrimp and Asparagus Stir-Fry

SERVES
3

Tester Rebecca said this made her think of "a tasty luncheon at a sweet little bistro in town." And if you have the Lemon Stir-Fry Sauce (see page 34) in the refrigerator, it will take you a big 10 minutes.

If the shrimp are wet, pat 'em dry with paper towels.

Snap the ends off the asparagus where they want to break naturally. Lay the remainder on your cutting board and cut them into 1-inch (2.5 cm) lengths.

Trim the roots from the scallions and then slice the white part about ¼ inch (6 mm) thick.

Put a wok or big skillet over the highest heat. Add half the lard or oil and let it get good and hot. Throw in the shrimp and stir-fry until they're pink clear through. Remove the shrimp to a plate and reserve. Add the rest of the lard or oil and let it get hot. Now add the asparagus and the scallions and stir-fry them until the asparagus is brilliantly green, no more. Dump the shrimp back into the pan and pour in the Lemon Stir-Fry Sauce. Stir to coat everything. Let it simmer for just a minute or two and then serve immediately.

1 pound (455 g) raw, shelled, medium-sized shrimp

1 pound (455 g) asparagus, not too thin

1 bunch of scallions

3 tablespoons (42 g) lard or coconut oil, divided

¼ cup (60 ml) Lemon Stir-Fry Sauce (See page 34.)

Per serving: 303 calories, 16 g fat, 33 g protein, 7 g carbohydrate, 2 g dietary fiber, 5 g net carbs

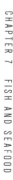

Mussels with White Wine Sauce

SERVES

4

4 pounds (1.8 kg) mussels

**1 batch White Wine Sauce
(See page 173.)**

Per serving: 643 calories, 33 g fat,
55 g protein, 19 g carbohydrate,
trace dietary fiber, 19 g net carbs

*Please note: Because the White Wine Sauce has only four
ingredients, this has five. Figure 1 pound (455 g) of mussels
per customer. Mussels are often farmed these days. If you
can get wild-caught clams instead, the same preparation will
work nicely.*

First things first: Tap each mussel to see if it closes. Any that
remain fearlessly open should be discarded. You can't be too
careful with shellfish.

Put a few inches (7.5 to 10 cm) of water on to boil in a pot that
will fit a steamer and has a tight lid.

Pull the "beard," the little clump of fibrous stuff, off the side
of each mussel. (Hands work fine for this.) Now dispatch your
mussels: Dump them in the steamer, and, whistling *Taps*, slap
on a lid. Steam the mussels for 10 minutes. Make your White
Wine Sauce in the meanwhile.

Take a peek. Very likely, some of the mussels will be open, and
others will still be closed. Use tongs to pull out the open ones
and put 'em on a plate. Put the lid back on the pot and let the
rest steam for another 5 minutes. Repeat the removing of the
mussels that have opened. If you have to give the really stub-
born ones another 5 minutes, do so, but it's not likely. Turn off
the steamer. Discard any mussels that did not open.

Turn on the broiler and put the oven rack about 8 inches (20 cm)
below it.

When the mussels have cooled enough to handle, twist off
the empty half of the shell. Arrange the shells with the meat
in them in a roasting pan or pans. Spoon a little White Wine
Sauce into each shell, about ¼ teaspoon; use more if you're
using clams. Broil the mussels for about 5 minutes until sizzling.
Serve immediately.

note

These calorie and carb counts
assume that you'll eat all the
sauce, which is unlikely.

Bacon and Bay Scallops

That Nice Boy I Married licked the plate clean. Yet this dish is rocket-fast and dead easy to make. I did, indeed, use bay scallops. They're far cheaper than sea scallops, and they cook quicker.

Put a big, heavy skillet over medium-low heat and start the bacon cooking. You want it crisp.

In the meanwhile, drain any liquid off of the scallops and use paper towels to pat them dry.

When the bacon is crisp, remove it to a plate and reserve. Toss the scallops in the bacon grease. Sauté the scallops quickly, sprinkling in the seafood seasoning ¼ teaspoon at a time as you stir and turn them. (This assures more even distribution of the seasoning than simply dumping it all in at once.)

If your scallops were wet-packed like mine, a bit more liquid will cook out of them. Let the scallops continue cooking for a few minutes until the liquid cooks down a little. (You want it to be a little thinner than cream.)

Plate the scallops. Crumble the bacon pretty fine or snip it up with your kitchen shears (my choice) and divide it between the plates. Snip the parsley over each and then serve immediately.

4 slices of bacon

1 pound (455 g) bay scallops

1 teaspoon seafood seasoning, such as Old Bay

1 tablespoon (4 g) minced fresh parsley

Per serving: 273 calories, 8 g fat, 42 g protein, 5 g carbohydrate, trace dietary fiber, 5 g net carbs

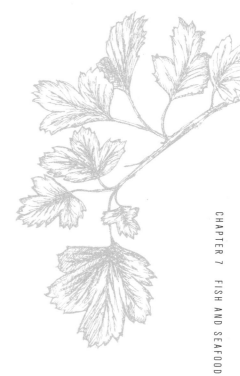

CHAPTER 7 FISH AND SEAFOOD

Lemon Tarragon Clams

SERVES 2

I wanted to make clams for That Nice Boy I Married, who loves them, and I was meditating on what to do with them. I realized I had tarragon leftover from the Lemon Tarragon Chicken, and this recipe was born. Two servings assumes this is a main course.

Put a pot that will fit the clams, with about 1 inch (2.5 cm) of water in it, over a high burner and add a steamer if you have one. (It's not essential, but it keeps you from needing to drain 'em.) Bring the water to a rolling boil and then throw in your clams, murmuring an elegy as you send them to their doom. Slap on a good, tight lid. Steam the clams for 10 minutes.

In the meanwhile, combine the oil, lemon juice, tarragon, and garlic. Let it sit, flavors infusing, while the clams finish opening.

When the timer beeps, check to see if your clams are open. Chances are some will be, and others won't. Using tongs, fish out the open ones and put the lid back on. Let the rest continue steaming, checking every few minutes, until they've all opened and been removed. (In the unlikely event that you have one that simply will not open, toss it. Seafood, you know.)

Turn on the broiler and set the rack about 8 inches (20 cm) below.

When the clams have cooled enough to handle, twist off and discard the halves of the shells that don't have the meat in them. Arrange the meaty ones in your roasting pan. Spoon the oil/lemon/tarragon mixture over them, dividing it evenly, making sure to coat each bit of meat well.

Broil the clams for 3 minutes. When your timer beeps, rotate the pan to make sure everything cooks evenly and broil the clams for another 2 to 3 minutes. Pour any sauce that's escaped the shells back over them as you serve.

16 clams, alive in the shell

¼ cup (60 ml) extra-virgin olive oil

2 tablespoons (28 ml) lemon juice

1 tablespoon (4 g) fresh tarragon, minced

1 clove of garlic, crushed

Per serving: 331 calories, 28 g fat, 15 g protein, 5 g carbohydrate, trace dietary fiber, 5 g net carbs

Beef

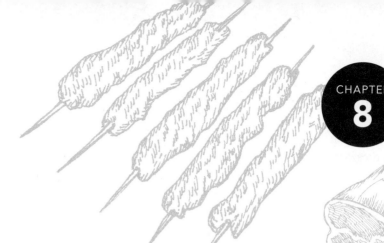

As the meat of grazing ruminants, beef goes back to our very earliest heritage. If you can afford it, grass-fed is nutritionally superior. It's also better for the environment than conventionally raised. If you have a deep freeze, buying a side of grass-fed beef, wrapped and ready for freezing, is the most affordable way to buy it.

However, I have it on good authority—Peter Ballerstaedt, a Ph.D. forage agronomist—that even most grain-finished beef is grazed for all but the last 4 to 6 weeks of its life. It's still nutritious stuff, and you know the family loves it.

Nose-to-Tail Burger

SERVES
40

This is the easiest way I know to get organ meats into your family's diet. Straight, this tastes a little stronger than plain ground chuck, but in chili, meat loaf, and the like you'd hardly know the difference, but your body will. Feel free to substitute this for the ground beef in any well-seasoned recipe. Don't tell your kids.

I'm counting all that meat as one ingredient because that's how you'll be getting it. Call up your local specialty butcher shop and ask them to grind all that stuff together for you. (Around here, grocery stores won't do this. I do have to go to my local specialty butcher shop, the wondrous Butcher's Block. A good butcher shop is a valuable resource.)

When you get the meat home, divide it into 5 batches of about 3 pounds (1.4 kg) each. Put a 3-pound (1.4 kg) chunk in a big mixing bowl, sprinkle 1 tablespoon each of the (7 g) gelatin and (9 g) bone meal over it, and use clean hands to squish it all together really well. If you have a stand mixer with dough hooks, use that instead.

As you get the gelatin and bone meal worked through a batch of meat, form it into burgers. (I make mine 6 ounces [170 g] each, which is where the 40-serving figure comes from.) Put a double layer of waxed paper between the burgers. Then work the gelatin and bone meal through the next batch, and so on.

Put the burgers in a few big snap-top containers and freeze. It will be easy to grab 18 ounces (510 g) of meat to make chili, meat loaf, or whatever. Feel free to use this in place of ground beef in just about any recipe.

12 pounds (5.5 kg) beef chuck

1 pound (455 g) beef liver

1 pound (455 g) beef heart

1 pound (455 g) beef tongue

5 tablespoons (35 g) unsweetened gelatin powder

5 tablespoons (45 g) bone meal

Per serving: 335 calories, 24 g fat, 27 g protein, 1 g carbohydrate, 0 g dietary fiber, 1 g net carbs

Five-Ingredient Chili!

Good chili has a lot of flavors, including onion, garlic, cumin, chili powder, oregano, and my secret ingredient, cocoa. That's six ingredients already. Here's salsa to the rescue.

In a big, heavy skillet over medium heat, start browning and crumbling the ground beef. When the pink is gone, pour off most of the fat. (We're not anti-fat, here; just looking not to have greasy chili.) Stir in everything else, rinsing out the salsa jar with the water to get the last bit of flavor. Bring the mixture to a simmer and let it cook for 20 minutes or so.

SERVES 3

1 pound (455 g) ground beef

1 jar (15½ ounces, [440 g]) chunky salsa

2 tablespoons (15 g) chili powder

½ tablespoon cocoa powder

1 tablespoon (3 g) dried oregano

½ of the salsa jar of water

Per serving: 532 calories, 42 g fat, 28 g protein, 13 g carbohydrate, 5 g dietary fiber, 8 g net carbs

note

If you'd like to keep all the fat in your chili, and with good grass-fed meat, it's a shame to lose any, you could add 8 ounces (225 g) of chopped mushrooms to the sautéing beef. They'll absorb the fat and add flavor, too.

Philippa's Meat Muffins

Philippa was my grandmother, and her meatloaf recipe is the one I grew up on. Here I've left out the dairy content, with no loss of flavor or texture. By cooking this in muffin tins, I've sliced a good 30 minutes off the cooking time. These reheat beautifully and are fab warmed up and served with fried eggs for breakfast.

Preheat the oven to 375°F (190°C or gas mark 5).

Do your usual meatloaf thing: Dump everything in a big mixing bowl and, using clean hands, smoosh it all together really well. Now make it into 9 rather large meatballs and drop one in each of 9 muffin tin hollows. (You can grease your muffin tin first, if you like. Mine is nonstick, so I didn't bother.) Bake the meatballs for 20 to 25 minutes and then serve them hot.

SERVES 9

18 ounces (510 g) ground chuck

1 medium onion, chopped fine

½ cup (50 g) pork rind crumbs

2 eggs

1 tablespoon (4 g) poultry seasoning

1 teaspoon salt

Per serving: 170 calories, 13 g fat, 11 g protein, 1 g carbohydrate, trace dietary fiber, 1 g net carbs

Bistro Burgers

SERVES
3

Here's your basic burger with just that extra nudge of flavor that makes it special. A nice sharp Cheddar or blue cheese would be good on these, if you're primal.

Plunk the ground chuck in a mixing bowl. Add the shallot, anchovies, mustard, salt, and pepper. Use clean hands to squish it all together really well. Now make three big patties. Keep them only ½ inch (1.3 cm) thick, no more. At this point, you can chill them for a while if it suits your convenience.

Put a big, heavy skillet over high heat. Let it get good and hot before you put the burgers in. Fry the burgers for 3 to 4 minutes per side, depending on how hot your stove gets and how well done you like your burgers. That's it!

1 pound (455 g) ground chuck

1 shallot, minced

2 anchovy fillets, minced

1 teaspoon spicy brown mustard

½ teaspoon salt

¼ teaspoon ground black pepper

Per serving: 410 calories, 32 g fat, 28 g protein, 1 g carbohydrate, trace dietary fiber, 1 g net carbs

note

Mince the shallot first and then your anchovies, or you'll be mincing your shallots on an oily, fishy cutting board.

Totally Inauthentic Machaca Eggs

SERVES
2

Huevos con Machaca are my favorite Mexican breakfast. I wanted to come up with similar recipe with far less work. Here it is! This would make a great quick supper, too.

Put a big, heavy skillet over medium heat and start browning and crumbling the ground beef. When the pink is gone from the meat, stir in the salsa. Keep cooking and stirring till most of the liquid has cooked away.

In a small bowl, scramble the eggs, stir them into the beef, and scramble till set.

12 ounces (340 g) ground beef

1 cup (260 g) hot or mild chunky salsa

4 eggs

Per serving: 695 calories. 54 g fat, 41 g protein, 9 g carbohydrate, 2 g dietary fiber, 7 g net carbs

Mega Food Stacks

This is a huge, seriously filling meal. And while I give you instructions here for caramelizing the onions, if you make the Slow Cooker Caramelized Onions on page 144, you can assemble these in about 10 minutes.

Start by caramelizing the onion: Put a big, heavy skillet over low heat. Melt 1 tablespoon (14 g) of the bacon grease and stir in the onion. Cook low and slow, stirring now and then, until the onion is limp and brown. (Don't burn 'em!)

Cook the bacon by your preferred method. (You could cook it before the onion and use the grease to cook them in, but that doesn't let you multitask. Anyway, you may have cleverly made caramelized onions in advance, and then you simply have to pull them out of your stash.)

Form the ground chuck into patties, keeping them about ½ inch (1.3 cm) thick.

Put another skillet (or the same skillet, cleaned, with the onion reserved) over high heat. Let it get good and hot and then throw in the burgers. Cook for 3 to 4 minutes, flip 'em, and cook for another 3 minutes.

Slice the cheese and cover each burger with slices. Cover the pan with a tilted lid, turn off the heat, and let the reserved heat melt the cheese.

While the cheese is melting, put yet another skillet over medium heat. Melt the rest of the bacon grease. When it's hot, crack in the eggs and cover the skillet. Keep a close eye on the eggs and cook them until the whites are set and the yolks are still runny.

Okay, start assembling your stacks: cheeseburger, covered with caramelized onions, topped with bacon that's been snapped in half and cross-hatched, topped with a fried egg. Serve immediately!

2 tablespoons (28 g) bacon grease, divided

1 small onion, thinly sliced

4 slices of bacon, cooked crisp

12 ounces (340 g) ground chuck

4 ounces (55 g) Cheddar cheese or other cheese (I used Kerrygold Derbyshire.)

2 eggs

Per serving: 955 calories, 78 g fat, 54 g protein, 6 g carbohydrate, 1 g dietary fiber, 5 g net carbs

Sriracha Steak

I made this with a nice, tender rib eye, but if you have a tougher cut, you could marinate it considerably longer. The acidity will help tenderize it. A well marinated chuck is a glorious thing.

Lay the steak in a nonreactive plate or baking dish—stainless steel, glass, or ceramic.

Run everything else through the blender until it's well combined.

Use a fork to stab the steak thoroughly all over. Now pour about one-third of the sriracha mixture over it and spread it to coat. Flip the steak and do the same on the other side with the second one-third of the sauce. Let this sit for 10 to 15 minutes, longer for a tougher cut.

Turn your broiler to high and set the oven rack close; I put mine on the top level. Oil your broiler pan or spray it with coconut oil cooking spray. Lay the steak on the broiler and slide it under the heat. The timing will depend a bit on the thickness of your steak and how well done you like it. (Mine was about 1 inch [2.5 cm] thick, and I gave it 7 minutes on the first side.) Flip the steak end-to-end. (This evens out cooking more than flipping it side-to-side.) Slide the steak back under the broiler. (I cooked mine for another 5 minutes.)

When the steak is done to your liking, put it on a plate or carving board and let it rest for 5 minutes. Pour the remaining one-third of the sauce over it, cut into portions, and serve immediately.

12 ounces (340 g) beef rib eye, sirloin, or strip

2 tablespoons (28 ml) sriracha

2 tablespoons (28 ml) lime juice

1 tablespoon (15 ml) fish sauce

3 cloves of garlic, crushed

Per serving: 470 calories, 37 g fat, 30 g protein, 5 g carbohydrate, trace dietary fiber, 5 g net carbs

note

I topped this with some chopped cilantro, but it's hardly essential, and I know many people aren't fond of it. Plus it is, of course, another ingredient. Suit yourself.

Slow Cooker Pike's Peak Roast

SERVES
12

Pike's Peak roast is a cut of beef round, and it's very lean. The marinade adds both flavor and fat. You have to start this a day ahead, but other than that, it's a snap.

In a big, non-reactive bowl—stainless steel, glass, or ceramic—combine the wine, oil, garlic, salt, and pepper. Plunk the roast in, and turn it once or twice to coat. Stick it in the fridge and forget about it till tomorrow, except to turn it over should you open the fridge and notice it.

Okay, it's tomorrow. Drain the roast, reserving the marinade. Put your big, heavy skillet over high heat and melt the bacon grease or lard. Sear the beef all over, until it is nice and brown.

When the roast is done searing, plunk it in a slow cooker. (I used my big 5½ quart (6 L) one. Pour the reserved marinade into the skillet and stir it around, dissolving all the nice brown stuff, and then pour it over the roast. Put on the lid, set it to low, and cook it for 8 hours or so.

That's it! Fish the roast out, carve it, and serve it with the pot liquid.

1 beef round roast (4 pounds, or 1.8 kg)

½ cup (120 ml) dry red wine

½ cup (120 ml) olive, avocado, or MCT oil

2 cloves of garlic

¼ teaspoon salt

¼ teaspoon ground black pepper

3 tablespoons (42 g) bacon grease or lard

Per serving: 425 calories, 32 g fat, 31 g protein, trace carbohydrate, trace dietary fiber, 0 g net carbs

note

I'd serve Fauxtatoes (see page 128) with this; they're good with the pot liquid. You can thicken the sauce with a little glucomannan if you want, but that's another step and ingredient.

Balsamic Pot Roast

SERVES
6

To make this dish hardier, chunk some turnips and add them to the slow cooker. Put them beneath the roast, or they'll be undercooked.

Put a big, heavy skillet over high heat. When it's hot, melt the bacon grease and start searing the chuck roast.

Measure the tomato sauce (unless you're using an 8-ounce [235 ml] can) and stir the vinegar into it.

When the chuck is completely browned, spread half of the shallot on the bottom of the slow cooker. Place the roast on top. Scatter the remaining shallot over the roast.

Pour the tomato sauce mixture into the skillet and stir it around, scraping up all of the tasty brown bits. Pour this sauce over the roast. Slap on the lid, set it to low, and let the whole thing cook for 7 to 8 hours.

1 tablespoon (14 g) bacon grease

1 beef chuck roast (2 pounds, or 900 g)

1 shallot, sliced paper thin

1 cup (245 ml) tomato sauce

2 tablespoons (28 ml) balsamic vinegar

Per serving: 349 calories, 26 g fat, 24 g protein, 4 g carbohydrate, 1 g dietary fiber, 3 g net carbs

Chipotle Pot Roast

SERVES
9

It's nice to serve Fauxtatoes (see page 128) with this.

In a big, heavy skillet over medium high heat, sear the chuck roast well on both sides in the bacon grease. Transfer the roast to your slow cooker.

Pour the stock into the skillet and stir it around, dissolving any nice brown bits. Stir in the salsa and then pour this mixture over the roast. Slap on the lid, set it to low, and let the whole thing cook for a good 6 to 8 hours.

Serve the beef with the sauce. If you feel like doing marginally more work, when the roast is done, you can put it on a platter and keep it warm while you transfer the sauce to a saucepan. Bring it to a low boil and let it cook down by about one-third. This intensifies the flavor, but it's not essential.

1 beef chuck roast (3 pounds, or 1.4 kg)

2 tablespoons (28 g) bacon grease

½ cup (120 ml) beef stock

1 cup (260 g) chipotle salsa

Per serving: 353 calories, 27 g fat, 25 g protein, 2 g carbohydrate, trace dietary fiber, 2 g net carbs

Balsamic Marinated Chuck

Don't be scared of papain; it's natural papaya enzyme. I bought a big sack of it through Amazon.com when I couldn't find meat tenderizer with no garbage added.

Lay the chuck on a rimmed plate and stab it viciously all over with a fork, venting your ire on both sides.

In a bowl, mix together everything else except the bacon grease. Spread half of the mixture on one side of the chuck, flip it, and spread the rest on the other side. Let it sit for 15 to 30 minutes.

Now put a big, heavy skillet over high heat. Melt the bacon grease and slosh it around. Throw in the chuck and cook it for about 5 minutes per side, depending on the thickness. Transfer the chuck to a platter and let it sit for 5 minutes before cutting it into portions and serving.

SERVES 3

1 beef chuck roast (1 pound, or 455 g), about ½ inch (1.3 cm) thick

2 tablespoons (28 ml) balsamic vinaigrette

2 teaspoons coconut aminos

1 teaspoon spicy brown mustard

Scant ¼ teaspoon papain

1 tablespoon (14 g) bacon grease or other fat

Per serving: 406 calories, 33 g fat, 24 g protein, 1 g carbohydrate, trace dietary fiber, 1 g net carbs

Pesto Chuck

Chuck is tough but flavorful. The trick is to marinate or otherwise tenderize it. This created a tender and super tasty steak.

Using a fork, stab the chuck to create punctures every ¼ inch (0.6 cm) or so.

In a bowl, stir together the Meat Tenderizer and pesto, mixing well. Spread this evenly all over both sides of the chuck. Throw it in the fridge and go to work.

At T-minus-7-minutes-and-counting to supper, put a big, heavy skillet over highest heat. When it's hot, throw in the bacon grease, slosh it around, and then throw in the chuck. I cooked mine for 3 minutes on one side, and 4 minutes on the other, and it came out crusty brown on the outside and pink in the middle. Yum.

SERVES 3

1 beef chuck roast (1 pound, or 455 g), about ½ inch (1.3 cm) thick

½ tablespoon Meat Tenderizer (See page 36.)

1 tablespoon (15 g) pesto sauce

1 tablespoon (14 g) bacon grease

Per serving: 380 calories, 30 g fat, 25 g protein, trace carbohydrate, trace dietary fiber, 0 g net carbs

Beef and Broccoli Stir-Fry

This is a simple, family-pleasing stir-fry. It's up to you whether you want to use fresh broccoli or frozen. If you use frozen, choose what's labeled "broccoli cuts." These are bigger than chopped, but smaller than spears. Frozen broccoli will need less steaming than fresh.

Slice the beef into thin strips. (Having the meat halfway frozen makes this easier.) Put it in a bowl and stir in the Basic Stir-Fry Sauce.

If you're using fresh broccoli, cope with that next. Whack off the stems and use a paring knife to peel off the tough skin. Now cut the stem and the florets into evenly sized bites. Steam them till they're brilliantly green, but not quite tender.

Slice the onion into half rounds about ¼ inch (6 mm) thick and separate them.

Drain the beef strips, reserving the marinade. Put them on a couple of layers of paper towels for a minute or two to absorb the moisture. (This reduces splattering.) Drain the steamed broccoli, too.

Okay, is everything prepped? You're ready to cook. Put a wok or big skillet over medium heat and add 1 tablespoon (14 g) of the lard or oil. Add the walnuts, stir them until they smell toasty, remove them from the pan to a plate, and reserve.

Add another tablespoon (14 g) or so of fat to the pan and crank the heat up as high as it will go. Throw in the beef and stir-fry till all the pink is gone. Remove the beef from pan to a plate, and reserve.

Add the rest of the fat to the pan and throw in the onion and broccoli. Stir-fry it until tender-crisp. Return the beef to the skillet and add the reserved marinade. Stir it all up and then let it cook until the marinade has cooked down about halfway. Stir in the walnuts and serve immediately.

1 pound (455 g) beef round

¼ cup (60 ml) Basic Stir-Fry Sauce (See page 33.)

2 pounds (900 g) broccoli

½ of a large onion

¼ cup (30 g) chopped walnuts

¼ cup (56 g) lard or bland coconut oil

Per serving: 454 calories, 33 g fat, 29 g protein, 12 g carbohydrate, 5 g dietary fiber, 7 g net carbs

note

If you have grain-eaters in the family, or you're a devotee of Paul Jaminet's "safe starches," you can serve rice with this. Me, I eat it straight. Safe starches aren't so safe for those of us with lousy carb metabolisms.

Bulgogi Skewers

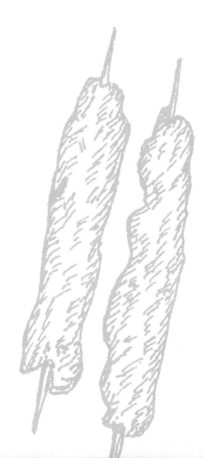

SERVES 4

As Korean-ish skewered beef, this is quick and easy to make. While this assumes it's a main dish, you can make these smaller and serve them as pick-up food at a party. Even making the seasoning sauce, this is only five ingredients. You'll need eight skewers for this. If they're metal, you're good. If they're bamboo, you'll have to remember to put them in to soak in the morning or for at least a half hour before cooking time.

Cut the steak across the grain into thin strips. (This is easier if it's halfway frozen.) Throw the strips in a zipper-lock bag, pour in the sauce, and seal, pressing out the air as you go. Turn the bag a few times to make sure all of the strips are coated. Throw it in the fridge and let them sit for at least a few hours. While you're at work is perfect.

Is it dinner time? Turn on the broiler or fire up the grill. Grab 8 skewers. Pull the bag out of the fridge and drain the marinade off into a bowl.

Thread the beef on the skewers, bending it back and forth, accordion-fashion.

Broil the skewers 6 to 8 inches (15 to 20 cm) from the heat or grill them, brushing them with the reserved marinade when you turn them. (If your broiler is like mine, you may want to turn your broiler pan end-to-end at this point to encourage more even cooking.) They shouldn't take more than 5 or 6 minutes.

In the meanwhile, stir the sesame seeds in a dry skillet over medium-low heat until they start to smell toasty. When the beef is done, plate the skewers, sprinkle the sesame seeds over them, and serve immediately.

1 beef round steak (1 pound, or 455 g)

Korean-ish Seasoning Sauce (See page 170.)

2 tablespoons (16 g) sesame seeds

Per serving: 263 calories, 12 g fat, 27 g protein, 10 g carbohydrate, 1 g dietary fiber, 9 g net carbs

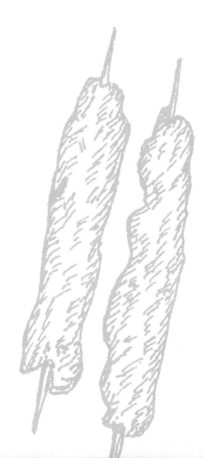

CHAPTER 8 BEEF

99

Venison Stew

The only part of this slow cooker stew that takes any time is browning the meat. Other than that? Cut stuff up and throw i[...] the pot. Let it cook all day. Dinner! Feel free to make this with[...] if you don't have a source of venison. I'd go with chuck or arr[...]

Season the venison cubes all over with salt and pepper.

Put a big, heavy skillet over medium heat and add 2 table[...] (28 ml) of the bacon grease. Get the grease hot and add venison cubes. Don't crowd them! They won't brown if y[...] do. Just resign yourself to the fact that you're going to [...] brown them in 5 or 6 batches.

While the venison is browning, peel the sweet potatoes and cut 'em in a ½-inch (1.3 cm) dice. Put 'em in the bottom of the slow cooker. Do the same with the onions, putting them on top of the sweet potatoes. During the time you're doing this, you'll need to flip the venison cubes and likely even remove the first batch to a plate and start a second batch browning. Add more bacon grease, a tablespoon (14 g) or so at a time, as you add more venison cubes.

When all the venison cubes are browned, dump all of them on top of the veggies in your slow cooker.

Pour the water into the skillet, using a bit of it to rinse off the plate you've been stashing venison cubes on, too. Crush the garlic into the water and add the oregano. Stir the whole thing around, scraping up all the yummy browned stuff on the skillet. Pour this over everything in the slow cooker. Slap the lid on, set it to low, and let it cook on low for 8 hours, or, if you're in a hurry, 4 to 5 hours on high.

1 tablespoon (\[...\] g) oregano

Per serving: 406 calories, 21 g fat, 36 g protein, 15 g carbohydrate, 2 g dietary fiber, 13 g net carbs

Pork and Lamb

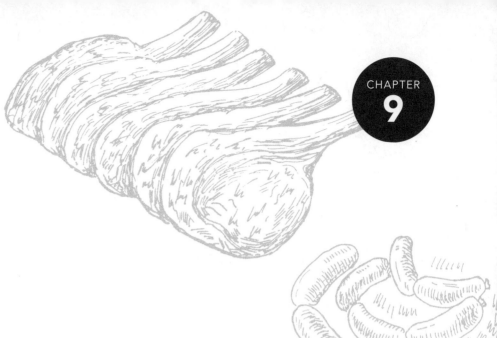

This is a really big chapter. I love pork in every form, and I consider the common belief that it is unhealthful to be slander. Pork steaks are quick and easy, pork shoulder is one of the best cuts for the slow cooker, and ribs are pure heaven.

So I wound up with a lot of pork recipes. As for lamb, you need to eat more of it. It is virtually all grass-fed, making it the only grass-fed meat in many American grocery stores. I find it puzzling that this country eats so little lamb. The rest of the world appreciates it thoroughly.

Apple-y Pork Steak

SERVES
2

Why I didn't think of this the moment I invented the Apple-y Dressing, I don't know. It's glaringly obvious. Apples and pork are a classic combination.

If you think of it early, great: Put the pork steak in a resealable bag and add 2 tablespoons (28 ml) of the dressing. Seal the bag, pressing out the air as you go. Turn and squeeze the bag until the pork is evenly covered with the dressing. Throw the bag in the fridge and let it cool its heels for a few hours.

If you think of it at the last minute, just lay the pork on a plate, spread 1 tablespoon (15 ml) of dressing over it, flip it, and spread another tablespoon (15 ml) on the other side. Give it 15 to 20 minutes.

Either way, when cooking time comes, the drill is simple and obvious: Put your skillet over medium heat. When it's good and hot, melt the bacon grease, slosh it around, and then throw in the pork steak. (Mine was about ½ inch [1.3 cm] thick, and I cooked it for about 8 minutes per side.)

Remove the steak. Add the water to the skillet and stir it around, dissolving the nice brown stuff. Now pour in the rest of the dressing. Let it simmer, stirring, for a minute or two. Cut the steak into 2 portions and plate. Pour the sauce over the top and serve immediately.

**1 pork shoulder steak
(1 pound, or 455 g)**

¼ cup (60 ml) Apple-y Dressing, divided (See page 32.)

1 tablespoon (14 g) bacon grease

2 tablespoons (28 ml) water

Per serving: 626 calories, 55 g fat, 29 g protein, 1 g carbohydrate, trace dietary fiber, 1 g net carbs

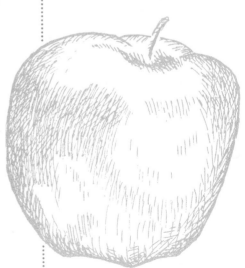

Pork Steak with Peppers and Onions

SERVES
2

With both a protein and a vegetable, this could stand as a complete meal, although a green salad would also go nicely.

Put a big, heavy skillet over high heat. Throw in the bacon grease and let it melt while you sprinkle both sides of the pork steak liberally with Creole Seasoning.

When the skillet's good and hot, throw in the steak. Cook the steak for 4 minutes. Flip the steak and cook it for 4 minutes on the other side. (If it's curling a little at the edge, just cut into it a little. I snip with my kitchen shears.)

Remove the now nicely browned pork steak to a plate and throw the pepper and onion into the skillet. Sauté, scraping up all of the nice brown stuff off the bottom of the skillet as you stir. As the pepper and onion start to soften, add the water and stir that in, too, again, scraping the brown stuff off of the bottom of the skillet.

Turn the burner down to medium low, spread out the peppers and onions, and lay the pork steak on top, pouring in any juices that accumulated on the plate. Cover the skillet and cook the pork for 10 minutes.

Serve the pork with the peppers and onions on top. A little parsley snipped on top is nice, but not essential.

2 tablespoons (28 g) bacon grease

1 pork shoulder steak (12 ounces, or 340 g)

Creole Seasoning (See page 35.)

½ of a large green pepper, cut into strips

¼ of a large onion, sliced

1 tablespoon (15 ml) water

Parsley (optional)

Per serving: 433 calories, 36 g fat, 22 g protein, 3 g carbohydrate, 1 g dietary fiber, 2 g net carbs

note

If you're a chili head, you could add a hot pepper to this.

Pork Steak with Grapefruit and Thyme

I love pork shoulder steaks! They're quick, easy, tasty, cheap, and endlessly variable. The grapefruit adds a fresh, bright tang. This calls for ¼ of a grapefruit. I will assume you will either make another grapefruit recipe soon or simply eat the leftover ¾ grapefruit. You could double this recipe and use half of a grapefruit, but my skillet won't fit two pork steaks this size.

Put a big, heavy skillet over medium heat. In the meanwhile, season the pork steak with salt and pepper on both sides.

When the skillet is good and hot, melt the bacon grease, slosh it around to cover the bottom of the skillet, and throw in the steak. Cook the steak for 7 to 8 minutes on each side until it is nice and brown, and, of course, done through.

When the steak is done, remove it to a plate. Throw the onion in the skillet and sauté it for a couple of minutes. Now squeeze in the grapefruit juice, getting every drop. Add the thyme, and stir it all up, scraping the nice brown stuff off the bottom of the skillet as you go.

Put the steak back in the skillet, turning to coat both sides. Let it simmer in the grapefruit mixture for just a minute or two, as it reduces. Then plate the steak, scrape everything from the skillet over it, and serve.

1 pork shoulder steak
(12 ounces, or 340 g)

Salt and ground black pepper,
to taste

1 tablespoon (14 g) bacon
grease

3 tablespoons (30 g) minced red
onion

¼ of a pink grapefruit

¼ teaspoon dried thyme

Per serving: 377 calories, 30 g fat,
22 g protein, 4 g carbohydrate,
1 g dietary fiber, 3 g net carbs

Apricot Pork Steak

SERVES
2

Fruit of every kind goes well with pork. You can find unsulfured dried apricots at your health food store. Be aware that they will not be a pretty orange color, but brown. S'okay, they're still apricots.

Put the apricots in a bowl and pour the boiling water over them. Let them rehydrate while you're cooking.

Put a big, heavy skillet over medium-high heat. In the meanwhile, season the pork steak with salt and pepper on both sides. Throw it in the skillet and brown it on both sides for about 5 minutes per side.

When the pork is getting brown, dump the apricots and water in your blender or food processor, along with the vinaigrette and mustard. Run it till you have a rough sauce. Pour the sauce over the pork, flipping it once or twice to coat. Cover the skillet with a tilted lid and turn the burner down to medium-low. Let it simmer for another 5 minutes or so, and the sauce will thicken. Plate the pork, scraping all the sauce from the skillet over the steak. Carve it into servings.

4 whole dried apricots or 8 halves

¼ cup (60 ml) boiling water

1 pork shoulder steak (1 pound, or 455 g)

Salt and ground black pepper, to taste

2 teaspoons lard or other fat

¼ cup (60 ml) White Balsamic Vinaigrette (See page 31.)

2 teaspoons spicy brown mustard

Per serving: 619 calories, 51 g fat, 30 g protein, 10 g carbohydrate, 1 g dietary fiber, 9 g net carbs

note

Do this with pork chops, if you prefer.

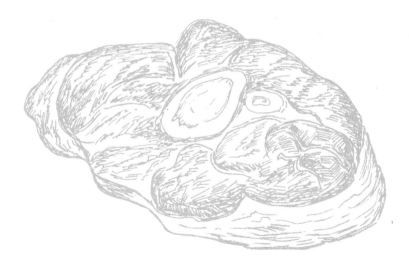

Lemon-Caper Pork Steak

SERVES 2

Is it obvious that shoulder steaks are my favorite cut of pork? They're much juicier and fattier than loin chops, and they're less expensive to boot. You can see why I'm always looking for new things to do with them!

Put a big, heavy skillet over medium heat. (Do this first, so it's hot when the steak hits the pan.)

Season the steak on both sides with salt and pepper. When the pan is hot, melt the lard, slosh it around to coat the pan, and throw in the steak. Let the steak cook till browned on the first side, flip it, and cook the other side till brown, too. Poke it right near the bone to see if the juices are running clear. If they're still pink, give it another couple of minutes.

When the steak is done, remove it to a platter. Leave the skillet over the heat, but turn it down a little. Squeeze in the juice from the lemon, getting every drop. Throw in the capers and add the garlic and hot sauce. Stir this all around, scraping up any nice brown stuff from the skillet. Scrape every bit of this mixture over the steak, cut it into servings, and devour.

1 pork shoulder steak (1 pound, or 455 g)

Salt and ground black pepper, to taste

1 tablespoon (14 g) lard or other fat

½ of a lemon

2 tablespoons (17 g) capers, minced

1 clove of garlic, crushed

1 teaspoon hot sauce, such as Frank's Hot Sauce, or to taste

Per serving: 467 calories, 37 g fat, 30 g protein, 2 g carbohydrate, trace dietary fiber, 2 g net carbs

notes

A little minced fresh parsley would be good here, but it's hardly necessary. This has a great big flavor as it is. This would work well with chicken, too—thighs, breasts, or both.

5-4-3-2 Ribs

SERVES 4

Note the measurements on the ingredients: 5-4-3-2! And this is mighty tasty, too.

Preheat the oven to 325°F (170°C or gas mark 3).

In a bowl, mix together everything but the ribs.

Lay the ribs in a roasting pan, preferably one with a cover. (I had to cut my slab up to fit it in my covered roaster.) If you don't have a roasting pan with a cover, foil works fine. Pour the seasoning mixture over the ribs. Cover, making sure the foil is sealed around the edges if that's what you're using, and roast the ribs for 30 minutes.

Uncover the ribs, flip them, basting to make sure all surfaces are coated, and re-cover. Roast the ribs for another 30 minutes.

Now's where a little judgment is called for because how done your ribs are getting will depend upon how thick your slab is. Look at them! Are they starting to pull away from the bone? Poke them with a fork. Do they feel tender? If they're still underdone, flip them, baste, and roast them for another 15 to 30 minutes. If they're getting there, go on to the next step.

Uncover the ribs, baste them well, and make sure they're meaty side up. Roast them for a final 10 to 15 minutes to reduce the liquid in the pan.

Pull the ribs out, let them cool for 5 minutes, and then cut them into individual ribs with your kitchen shears.

5 tablespoons (75 ml) water

¼ cup (60 ml) coconut aminos

3 tablespoons (45 ml) dry sherry

2 tablespoons (28 ml) white balsamic vinegar

3 pounds (1.4 kg) pork spareribs

Per serving: 633 calories, 50 g fat, 36 g protein, 4 g carbohydrate, 0 g dietary fiber, 4 g net carbs

Breakfast Sausage

SERVES
36

"Wait!" I hear you cry. "Not counting salt and pepper, this has six ingredients!" Ah, but you're going to have the butcher grind the pork shoulder and the fat together for you, so they actually count as one. This recipe makes quite a lot, too.

If you can make meat loaf, you can make this sausage! You'll need a grocery store that has actual people working behind the meat counter, though. Have the nice meat people grind 2½ pounds (1.1 kg) of pork shoulder with ½ pound (225 g) of pork fat. (You may need to ask them in advance, so that they save trimmed pork fat for you.) Take the nice fatty pork home and throw it in a big ol' bowl. Peel the shallots, drop them in your food processor, and pulse them until they're minced quite fine. Dump them in with the meat.

Add everything else. Now use clean hands to squish everything together very, very well. Congratulations! You now have sausage meat.

If you like, you can pan-fry a tiny bit of the mixture to see if you want to add more of this or that. Or you can just trust my palate. Either way, put the mixture in a big snap-top container and refrigerate it overnight to let the flavors blend.

Form into 36 patties of about 1⅓ ounces (38 g) each and freeze with waxed paper between them. (Here's a lesson from my mom: A double layer of waxed paper makes sausage patties —or hamburgers, or anything else you freeze this way—a lot easier to separate than a single layer. It's easiest to just fold a strip in half.)

2½ pounds (1.1 kg) pork shoulder

½ pound (225 g) pork fat

3 shallots

4 teaspoons (22 g) salt

4 teaspoons (3 g) dried sage, rubbed

1 tablespoon (20 g) maple syrup

1 tablespoon (15 g) spicy brown mustard

2 teaspoons ground black pepper

Per serving: 99 calories, 9 g fat, 5 g protein, 1 g carbohydrate, trace dietary fiber, 1 g net carbs

Easy Pulled Pork

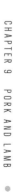

SERVES 12

I cannot think of an easier or better way to feed a crowd than this. Any time the whole gang is coming to your house, this, along with a vat of slaw, should be your front-line consideration. Provide buns for people who actually eat—ugh!—gluten, and they won't even figure out your scheme.

Using a carving fork, ruthlessly stab the pork shoulder all over. (Think of that kid who was really, really mean to you in eighth grade and go for it.) Smear the mustard all over the roast, covering every surface.

In a bowl, mix together the paprika, chili powder, and garlic powder. Sprinkle this mixture liberally over the whole surface of your pork as well. If you have any left over—I did—save it. It comes in handy for playing with the leftovers.

Drop the roast in a big ol' slow cooker, slap on the lid, and set it to low. Let it cook for 12 hours or so. When the pork is falling-off-the-bone tender, use two forks to shred it, mixing it into the liquid that will have accumulated in the pot. Fish out the bones with tongs.

1 pork shoulder (5 pounds, or 2.2 kg)

¼ cup (60 g) spicy brown mustard

1 tablespoon (17 g) paprika, hot smoked

1 tablespoon (8 g) chili powder

1 teaspoon garlic powder

Per serving: 344 calories, 26 g fat, 25 g protein, 1 g carbohydrate, trace dietary fiber, 1 g net carbs

Throwback Slow Cooker Luau

SERVES 12

This is very mid-twentieth century. It's super-simple, awfully good, cheap, and serves a crowd. What more could you want from a recipe? All of my local grocery stores sell containers of fresh pineapple chunks. I can watch them cut 'em up, so I know there's no junk added.

This is so easy! Plunk the roast in a slow cooker, fatty side up.

Run everything else through your food processor until the pineapple is pulverized. Pour the mixture evenly all over the roast. Slap on the lid, set it to low, and go do something else for a good 14 hours or so.

1 pork shoulder roast
(5 pounds, or 2.3 kg)

1 cup (240 g) Dana's Paleo
Ketchup (See page 30.)

6 ounces (170 g) fresh pineapple
chunks

¼ cup (60 ml) coconut aminos

Per serving: 364 calories, 26 g fat,
25 g protein, 7 g carbohydrate,
1 g dietary fiber, 6 g net carbs

Broccoli-Pepper Skillet Supper

SERVES 3

Want this recipe to be even quicker and easier than it already is? When you buy the bag of broccoslaw, grab peppers and onions from the grocery store salad bar.

Halve the pepper lengthwise and remove the core. Cut it crosswise, too, and then into thin strips. Peel the onion and slice it thinly, lengthwise. Cube or slice the pork into bite-sized pieces.

Put a big, heavy skillet over medium-high heat, melt 1 tablespoon (8 g) of the lard, and sauté the pork until all of the pink is gone. Remove the pork from the skillet.

Melt the rest of the lard and throw in the broccoslaw, pepper, and onion. Toss till it's all coated with fat. Cover the skillet and let the whole thing cook for 3 to 4 minutes. Toss again, re-cover, and cook it for another 3 to 4 minutes. Do it one more time. Now taste a broccoli sliver. Is it getting tender?

Stir in the vinaigrette, re-cover, and cook the whole thing for another few minutes. Make sure the veggies are tender-crisp, stir in the pork, and serve.

1 red bell pepper

1 onion

12 ounces (340 g) boneless pork
sirloin

2 tablespoons (28 g) lard or
other fat, divided

1 bag (12 ounces, or 340 g) of
broccoslaw

⅓ cup (80 ml) vinaigrette
(You can use balsamic, Italian,
or whatever is in your fridge.)

Per serving: 410 calories, 30 g fat,
26 g protein, 10 g carbohydrate,
4 g dietary fiber, 6 g net carbs

Billy Joe

One of the recipes I have repeated most often is Joe, made with browned ground beef, spinach, and eggs. This version with pulled pork and cabbage struck me as kind of Southern, hence the name.

In a big skillet over medium heat, sauté the onion and cabbage in the bacon grease. Turn the vegetables often. When they're softened and getting flecks of brown, stir in the pulled pork. Let it heat through. Mix it all up, so the vegetables and meat get well acquainted.

In a bowl, scramble the eggs and then pour 'em into the skillet and stir till they're set. Season the eggs with salt and pepper.

SERVES 5

1 medium onion, finely diced

½ head savoy cabbage, thinly sliced

¼ cup (56 ml) bacon grease

1½ cups (350 g) leftover Easy Pulled Pork (See page 109.)

5 eggs

Salt and ground black pepper, to taste

Per serving: 325 calories, 26 g fat, 18 g protein, 3 g carbohydrate, 1 g dietary fiber, 2 g net carbs

Coffee-Rubbed Pork Chops

Coffee-rubbed meat is kinda trendy, and with good reason. It adds a lovely dark, rich flavor. This is quick and easy, too.

In a bowl, combine the coffee, erythritol, salt, chili powder, and paprika. Rub both sides of the pork chops liberally with this mixture.

Put your biggest heavy skillet over medium heat. Let it get good and hot.

Throw in the bacon grease and slosh it about as it melts to coat the bottom of the skillet. Now throw in the chops. The cooking time will depend on the thickness of your chops. (Mine were about ½ inch [1.3 cm] thick, and they took about 7 minutes per side. If your chops are thicker than mine, turn down the burner a bit and cover the skillet with a tilted lid to reflect heat back at the chops. This way you can cook them through before they're scorched on the outside. Browned is good; scorched is bad.)

SERVES 4

2 tablespoons (10 g) coffee, espresso ground

1 tablespoon (12 g) erythritol or Sucanat

2 teaspoons salt

1 teaspoon chili powder

1 teaspoon hot smoked paprika

4 pork chops (6 ounces, or 170 g each)

1 tablespoon (14 g) bacon grease

Per serving: 296 calories, 20 g fat, 26 g protein, 1 g carbohydrate, trace dietary fiber, 1 g net carbs

Mirepoix Pork Chops

Mirepoix is a classic French seasoning mixture of sautéed onion, carrot, and celery. It's great with many things. Here, it makes these pork chops quite special. Fauxtatoes (see page 128) are good with this to catch the extra sauce.

Put a big, heavy skillet over medium-high heat.

Season the chops with salt and pepper and start browning them in 1 tablespoon (14 g) of the bacon grease.

In the meanwhile, peel the onion and carrot and cut them and the celery into chunks. Drop them in your food processor and pulse till everything is chopped fine.

Turn the chops! When the chops are browned on both sides, remove them to a plate.

Melt the rest of the bacon grease and add the vegetable mixture. Sauté until it's turned limp and started to brown. Now stir in the broth.

Put the chops back into the skillet, turning to acquaint both sides with the mirepoix. Settle them down into the mixture. Turn the heat down to a simmer, cover the skillet, and let the whole thing cook for 20 to 25 minutes or until the chops are done through.

Serve with the mirepoix spooned over the chops.

3 pork chops (6 ounces, or 170 g each)

Salt and ground black pepper, to taste

2 tablespoons (28 g) bacon grease, divided

½ of a medium onion

1 medium carrot

1 medium rib of celery

½ cup (120 ml) chicken broth

Per serving: 367 calories, 26 g fat, 28 g protein, 5 g carbohydrate, 1 g dietary fiber, 4 g net carbs

Peach-and-Picante Pork Chops

SERVES 3

This is an interesting and yummy combination. You can double this recipe if you like, but you'll need a bigger skillet than mine. Whether you'll need liquid stevia extract or not will depend very much upon your peaches. If they're ripe and sweet, you won't need it. If they're a bit less so, you'll probably want it.

Put a big, heavy skillet over medium-high heat and melt the bacon grease. When it's hot, season the chops with salt and pepper and throw them in the skillet. Brown the chops for 3 to 4 minutes per side.

In the meanwhile, run the salsa, peaches, and water through your blender or food processor. (I quit when the sauce was still a little rough because I like it that way.)

Remove the browned chops from the skillet and park them on a plate for a minute.

Pour the sauce into the skillet and stir it around, scraping up any tasty brown stuff. Now settle the chops back down into it, flipping the chops once to coat both sides.

Cover the skillet, turn the burner down to low, and let the whole thing simmer for 15 to 20 minutes. Taste the sauce. If it needs to be a tiny bit sweeter, add 2 or 3 drops of stevia and stir it in. Serve the chops with the sauce, of course.

1 tablespoon (14 g) bacon grease

3 pork chops (6 ounces, or 170 g each)

Salt and ground black pepper, to taste

½ cup (130 g) salsa

½ cup (85 g) diced peaches

¼ cup (60 ml) water

Lemon–flavored liquid stevia extract (optional)

Per serving: 363 calories, 29 g fat, 22 g protein, 3 g carbohydrate, 1 g dietary fiber, 2 g net carbs

note

If I were going to add anything to this, it would be a little extra cilantro and hot sauce. But then, I like cilantro and hot sauce in just about anything.

Pork Chops with Apples and Sage

SERVES
4

When I was a kid, my mom always served applesauce with pork chops. That's what inspired this dish.

Preheat the oven to 325°F (170°C or gas mark 3). Grease a baking dish big enough for the chops.

Put a big, heavy skillet over medium heat. While it's heating, season the chops with salt and pepper on both sides.

Melt the bacon grease and start the chops browning. You'll need at least 5 minutes per side, and you may need to cook them in two batches.

In the meanwhile, peel and slice the apple and onion pretty thin. Lay them in the bottom of the baking dish. Okay, the chops are brown. Arrange them on the apples and onions.

In a bowl, stir together the broth and sage and pour the mixture over the chops. Cover with foil and then use a fork or knife tip to poke holes in it to let steam out.

Let the whole thing cook for 20 to 30 minutes. Check to see how wet the whole thing is. If the broth needs reducing, take the foil off and let it go another 10 minutes. Serve the chops with the apples, onions, and pan liquid on top.

4 pork chops (6 ounces, or 170 g each)

Salt and ground black pepper, to taste

2 tablespoons (28 g) bacon grease

1 apple

1 onion

1 cup (235 ml) chicken broth

4 teaspoons (3 g) dried sage

Per serving: 413 calories, 32 g fat, 23 g protein, 8 g carbohydrate, 2 g dietary fiber, 6 g net carbs

Pork and Peach Kebabs

SERVES
5

This dish is pretty and good! If you do all of the prep in advance, when you get home from work, all you have to do is skewer stuff and cook. Honestly, I don't think these need another thing except maybe a crisp green salad. You'll need five skewers for this. If they're metal, you're good. If they're bamboo, you'll have to soak them for at least a half hour before cooking time.

Cut the pork into cubes, aiming for 25 of 'em. Put them in a nonreactive bowl—stainless steel, glass, or ceramic—and pour ¼ cup (60 ml) of the Honey Mustard Dressing and Dipping Sauce over them. Stir to coat and then throw this in the fridge. Let it sit until you're ready to cook dinner. All day is fine, though if you're going to let it go that long, you might want to put it in a snap-top container.

Okay, dinner time is impending. Turn on your broiler to high and set the rack about 6 inches (15 cm) below it.

Peel and slice the peaches. (If you're using nectarines, there's no need to peel them.)

Whack the onion into chunks.

Now, grab 5 skewers and thread them thusly: pork cube, a piece of onion a couple leaves thick, and a peach slice. Repeat, ending with a pork cube.

Lay the skewers on the broiler pan and brush them with some of the remaining Honey Mustard dressing. Slide the skewers under the broiler and broil them for 5 minutes. Then turn the broiler pan end-to-end, in the interests of even cooking. Broil them for another 5 minutes.

When the timer beeps again, flip all of your skewers over and brush them with the last of the dressing. Do the same thing—broil them for 5 minutes, turn them end to end, and then broil them for 5 minutes more and serve.

1 boneless pork loin (2 pounds, or 900 g), cut about 1½ inches (3.2 cm) thick

⅓ cup (80 ml) Honey Mustard Dressing and Dipping Sauce, divided (See page 33.)

3 peaches or nectarines

1 medium onion

Per serving: 245 calories, 12 g fat, 24 g protein, 11 g carbohydrate, 2 g dietary fiber, 9 g net carbs

notes

Confession: I thought of this in December, when peaches were pretty thin on the ground. So I used frozen, unsweetened peach slices, and they worked beautifully.

The wintry birth of this recipe also explains why I cooked them under the broiler. In the summer, you certainly could cook these on your grill.

Stewed Lamb and Rutabaga

SERVES
4

This is peasant food at its best. If you like, you can use boneless stewing lamb, but the bones add flavor and nutrition. Anyway, what could be more Paleo? The prep for this is easy, but it takes a long time to cook. You might want to start the night before.

Preheat the oven to 350°F (180°C or gas mark 4).

Season the lamb bones with salt and pepper. Lay them in a metal roasting pan with the fattiest side up. Roast the lamb for 20 to 30 minutes, flip it, and then roast for another 20 minutes or so.

In the meanwhile, dice the onion and rutabaga into ½ inch (1.3 cm) bits. Dump 'em in the bottom of a slow cooker. (I used the standard 4-quart [3.8 L] model.)

When the bones are browned, place them on top of the vegetables. Pour the broth over it all and drop the bay leaves on top. Slap on the lid, set the slow cooker to low, and leave it for…well, a long time. Mine went 18 hours, and it was wonderful. Add more salt and pepper to taste. Remove the bay leaves before serving.

3 pounds (1.4 kg) meaty lamb neck bones if you can get 'em

Salt and ground black pepper, to taste

1 large onion

½ of a large rutabaga (Large is grapefruit-sized. You could use a baseball-sized one instead.)

½ cup (120 ml) strong chicken broth

2 bay leaves

Per serving: 722 calories, 57 g fat, 45 g protein, 4 g carbohydrate, 1 g dietary fiber, 3 g net carbs

Harissa Burgers

SERVES
3

Spicy and juicy, these are related to kofta, a favorite Middle Eastern street food.

Dump everything in a bowl and use clean hands to smoosh it together really well. Form the lamb into three patties, about ½ inch (1.3 cm) thick.

Put a big, heavy skillet over high heat. Let it get good and hot before you add the burgers. Cook the burgers for 3 to 4 minutes per side, depending on whether you like them pinker or less so. Serve the burgers immediately.

1 pound (455 g) ground lamb

1 tablespoon (16 g) harissa

2 tablespoons (20 g) minced onion

1 clove of garlic, crushed

Per serving: 435 calories, 36 g fat, 25 g protein, 2 g carbohydrate, trace dietary fiber, 2 g net carbs

Mythic Lamburgers

SERVES 3

Somewhere in the mists of time, a hunter killed a lamb and found cheese curds in its stomach. I'm betting he served the two together. Wouldn't you?

1 pound (455 g) ground lamb

1 tablespoon (11 g) Mediterranean seasoning (McCormick's makes this. It comes in a grinder, like a peppermill.)

6 tablespoons (56 g) feta cheese

3 tablespoons (21 g) chopped sun-dried tomatoes, packed in olive oil

Plunk the lamb in a mixing bowl. Now grind a tablespoonful (11 g) of the Mediterranean seasoning. Throw the seasoning in and use your hands to squish it through the lamb really well. Form the lamb into three patties, about ¾ inch (1.9 cm) thick.

Put a big, heavy skillet over medium-high heat and let it get hot before you lay your lamburgers in it. Cook them till they're brown on both sides, but not all dried out. (They should be a little pink in the center when you cut into them.)

In the meanwhile, crumble the feta and chop the sun-dried tomatoes. Top each burger with 2 tablespoons (19 g) feta, turn down the burner, and cover the skillet for 1 minute to let it melt a bit. Plate the burgers, topping the feta with the sun-dried tomatoes.

Per serving: 485 calories, 40 g fat, 28 g protein, 3 g carbohydrate, trace dietary fiber, 3 g net carbs

notes

I spotted McCormick's Gourmet Mediterranean Style Sea Salt Grinder at Costco, so I read the label. It contains sea salt, garlic, spices (including black pepper, fennel, rosemary, oregano, and basil), onion, red bell pepper, extractives of garlic, and extractives of paprika. Okay, so Ogg didn't have "extractives," but there are no grains, gluten, sugar, or soy. I pronounced it good, brought it home, and made these.

Lamb Steak with Ruby Grapefruit and Rosemary

SERVES
2

Watch for leg of lamb to go on sale in the spring. When you find a good price, have the nice meat guys slice one into steaks ½- to ¾-inch (1.3 to 1.9 cm) thick and stash them in the freezer. It's cheaper than lamb chops, and it's far quicker to cook than a whole leg. Plus you get a marrow bone in the middle of each as a bonus. Eat the marrow! It's like meat butter.

Put your big, heavy skillet over medium heat.

Sprinkle both sides of the lamb steak with Seasoned Salt and pepper. When the skillet is hot, melt the lard, slosh it around, and then throw in the steak. Sear it well on both sides. (If it starts to curl, grab kitchen shears and snip around the edges. This didn't happen to me, but it's been known to.)

While the lamb is browning, grab two bowls. Hold the half-grapefruit over one and use a small, sharp, thin-bladed knife to cut around each section, allowing the juice to drip into the bowl. Put the sections in the other bowl, removing any seeds. Squeeze all the juice from the empty rind into the juice bowl.

Somewhere in here, you'll flip your lamb steak, I assume. Anyway, when it's well browned on both sides, remove it to a plate. Turn the burner to low. Crush in the garlic and add the rosemary. Now pour in the juice and stir it around, dissolving all the nice brown crusty stuff on the pan.

Put the steak back in the skillet, flipping to coat. Dump the sections in next to it. Cover the skillet and let the whole thing simmer for 5 to 6 minutes.

When you uncover the skillet, the grapefruit sections will have magically melted down into the sauce, leaving only small bits. Transfer the steak back to the plate you already used, cut into portions, and serve with the pan liquid poured over top.

1 lamb leg steak (1 pound, or 455 g)

Seasoned Salt (See page 35.), to taste

Ground black pepper, to taste

1 tablespoon (14 g) lard

½ of a ruby red grapefruit

1 clove of garlic, crushed

¼ teaspoon ground rosemary or 1 teaspoon minced fresh rosemary

Per serving: 493 calories, 37 g fat, 33 g protein, 6 g carbohydrate, 1 g dietary fiber, 5 g net carbs

Lamb Ribs

There they were, listed on the chalkboard at the farmers' market. I had to try them! They're wonderful, and this seasoning complements them perfectly. I know this looks like more than five ingredients, but remember, the salt, pepper, water, and cooking fat don't count.

Preheat the oven to 325°F (170°C or gas mark 3).

Find a metal roasting pan the right size to fit your rack of lamb ribs. (Metal is important; it will help your ribs brown. A glass baking dish, such as Pyrex, won't.)

In a bowl, mix together the cumin, coriander, salt, and pepper. Sprinkle both sides of the ribs liberally with this mixture, leaving maybe half of it in the bowl. Lay the ribs in their pan and stick 'em in the oven. Roast the ribs for 30 minutes.

In the meanwhile, crush the garlic into the remaining spice mixture. Add the water and stevia and stir it all up. Now stir in the lard. This is your mopping sauce.

When the timer beeps, baste the ribs on both sides with the mopping sauce, turning them over as you do so. Set the timer for another 30 minutes and go check Facebook or something.

Once again— when the timer beeps, baste the ribs all over, flipping them in the process. Do this another couple of times till the fat is good and brown and crispy looking and the meat is drawing away from the bones. Cut the ribs into servings with your kitchen shears.

2 pounds (900 g) lamb ribs

2 teaspoons cumin

2 teaspoons ground coriander

1 teaspoon salt

¼ teaspoon ground black pepper

3 cloves of garlic, crushed

½ cup (120 ml) water

9 drops of lemon-flavored liquid stevia extract

¼ cup (56 g) lard, melted, or fat of your choice

Per serving: 992 calories, 95 g fat, 33 g protein, 2 g carbohydrate, trace dietary fiber, 2 g net carbs

notes

That calorie and fat count is inaccurate because you won't use up all of the mopping sauce. Still, my lamb ribs were gloriously fatty, and because lamb is virtually all grass-fed, that fat was seriously good for me. That's why the servings are pretty small. This is filling.

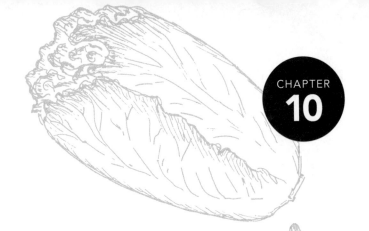

Side Salads

The simplest Paleo salad is fresh greens with one of the dressings in the Paleo Staples chapter on page 29. Throw in whatever is currently burgeoning in your garden, some fresh herbs, or a handful of toasted nuts or seeds, and it will be glorious.

Here, for your enjoyment, is a wide variety of salads. In particular, I've included a lot of salads that can be made ahead and stashed in the fridge. I love this sort of thing; it's tailor-made for busy lives. Knowing that your salad is waiting and all you need is a steak or a chop or a piece of fish is a real comfort when the errands are endless.

If I have a salad in the fridge, I'm likely to grab it for a snack, which is never a bad thing.

Be wary of bottled salad dressings. Even those sold in health food stores often contain canola or soy oils. See the Paleo Staples chapter for a selection of easy-to-make dressings that are guaranteed to please.

Winter Salad

I have always loved Waldorf salad, but there's a limit to how much apple my body can handle at one time. So I added those flavors to Caulirice (see page 128) and I swapped out Apple-y Dressing for the usual mayo. Yum!

Preheat the oven to 350°F (180°C or gas mark 4).

Trim the very bottom of the cauliflower stem and remove the leaves. Whack it into bits and run it through the shredding blade of a food processor. Now steam it for about 7 minutes.

While the cauliflower is steaming, spread the walnuts on a shallow baking sheet. Bake them for 5 minutes.

Pull the cauliflower off the heat, uncover, drain, and then dump it in a big mixing bowl. Let it cool for a few minutes before stirring in the celery, apple, and dressing. Season with salt and pepper and stir again.

SERVES 4

½ of a head of cauliflower

½ cup (60 g) chopped walnuts

1 cup (100 g) diced celery

1 cup (150 g) diced apple

1 cup (600ml) Apple-y Dressing (See page 32.)

Salt and ground black pepper, to taste

Per serving: 365 calories, 36 g fat, 6 g protein, 8 g carbohydrate, 3 g dietary fiber, 5 g net carbs

Classic Spinach Salad

This is a simple, old-school crowd pleaser. The yellow-and-white egg slices and red onion make it magazine pretty, too.

Dump the baby spinach in a big mixing bowl. Pour on the dressing and toss like mad till the spinach is all evenly coated. Pile the salad on four salad plates.

Top each salad with one egg, 1½ slices bacon, and 1 tablespoon (10 g) minced onion. Serve immediately because this doesn't hold well. (If you want to make this in advance, you can do the egg boiling and peeling, the bacon cooking, and the onion mincing as much as a day in advance. But once you dress the spinach, you need to follow through.)

SERVES 3

5 ounces (140 g) fresh baby spinach

1 cup (60 ml) Apple-y Dressing (See page 32.)

2 eggs, hard-boiled, peeled and sliced

3 slices of bacon, cooked and crumbled

2 tablespoons (20 g) minced red onion

Per serving: 316 calories, 29 g fat, 11 g protein, 5 g carbohydrate, 2 g dietary fiber, 3 g net carbs

Orange-y Spinach Salad

I've only used one orange here because I need to keep my carb count low. But if you like, feel free to add another orange's worth of segments to this.

First things first: Grate half of the zest off the orange and add it to the vinaigrette in a bowl. Whack the orange in half and squeeze the juice from half of it into the dressing, as well. Shake that up and let it sit while you assemble the salad.

Put the spinach in a big salad bowl. Slice the onion paper-thin, but don't put it in yet. Hold the remaining orange half over a small plate and use a small, thin, sharp knife to cut around each segment, freeing it. Cut those in half, making more but smaller bits.

Pour the dressing over the salad, pour in the juice from the plate with the orange segments, and toss very well. Arrange the onion and orange bits artistically on top and serve immediately.

1 navel orange

¼ cup (60 ml) Balsamic Vinaigrette (See page 31.)

10 ounces (280 g) fresh spinach

¼ of a red onion

Per serving: 60 calories, 5 g fat, 1 g protein, 2 g carbohydrate, 1 g dietary fiber, 1 g net carbs

Super Simple Slaw

I adore coleslaw, as anyone who has read my previous books knows. This version is super simple, yet quite wonderful. I kept thinking, "I could add ..." And then I'd think, "Nah. It's great the way it is."

Shred the cabbage and throw it in a big mixing bowl.

In another bowl, stir together the mayonnaise, vinegar, and mustard. Pour the dressing over the cabbage and toss till it's all evenly coated. That's it!

½ of a head of cabbage

½ cup (115 g) Good Ol' Mayonnaise (See page 30.)

1 tablespoon (15 ml) white balsamic vinegar

1 teaspoon spicy brown mustard

Per serving: 161 calories, 19 g fat, trace protein, 1 g carbohydrate, trace dietary fiber, 1 g net carbs

Beet and Orange Salad

SERVES
6

How pretty is this? This winter salad is a great reason to roast extra beets. With those and bagged salad, this is a snap. Tester Rebecca called this "incredible," and her husband dubbed it "fantastic." To do this the easiest way, see Slow Cooker Beets on page 145.

Preheat the oven to 350°F (180°C or gas mark 4).

Spread the walnuts on a shallow baking sheet and bake them for 6 to 7 minutes. (Set the timer or you'll be sorry!)

Slice the beets and place them in a bowl.

Hold the oranges over another bowl to catch the juice and halve them. Use a small, thin, sharp-bladed knife to cut around each section. Put these in yet one more bowl. (Don't panic. You can save on dishwashing by rinsing these bowls and using them to serve the salad.) Squeeze the juice remaining in the rinds into the juice bowl.

Mix the orange juice with the White Balsamic Vinaigrette.

By now, the oven timer has beeped. Pull out the walnuts and chop them.

Okay, you're ready to assemble! Pour ¼ cup (60 ml) of the dressing over the beets. Put the salad greens in a big salad bowl and pour the rest of the dressing over top. Toss like mad. Pile the greens into six bowls. Top each artistically with beets and orange sections and then a scattering of walnuts.

If you aren't feeding six people, only dress as many greens as you can use right away and then use the rest the next day.

⅓ cup (33 g) walnuts

3 medium beets, roasted

3 oranges

¾ cup (175 ml) White Balsamic Vinaigrette (See page 31.)

12 cups (660 g) mixed greens (Choose Italian blend or the like, something including arugula.)

Per serving: 260 calories, 20 g fat, 6 g protein, 19 g carbohydrate, 7 g dietary fiber, 12 g net carbs

note

Why not just toss everything with the dressing together? Because the beets will dye your oranges, and you won't get such pretty contrasting colors.

Hot Kickin' Curcubit Salad

SERVES 8

Did you know that melons and cucumbers are actually from the same family? They're curcubits. Here, two of your favorite curcubits team up to create a killer summer salad.

This is so easy! Place the watermelon, cucumber, and pepper in a bowl. Now wash your hands thoroughly, or you'll regret it the next time you touch your nose or eyes! Pour on the dressing and toss.

3 cups (450 g) diced watermelon

3 cups (405 g) diced cucumber

½ of a fresh jalapeño pepper

⅓ cup (80 ml) White Balsamic Vinaigrette (See page 31.)

Per serving: Total: 70 calories, 6 g fat, 1 g protein, 5 g carbohydrate, 1 g dietary fiber, 4 g net carbs

Apple-Maple Cucumber Salad

SERVES 4

Do look for unwaxed cucumbers. Organic cucumbers may be waxed with plant-sourced waxes, but conventionally grown cukes may well have synthetics, even petroleum-based waxes.

Scrub the cucumbers. If they're big, halve or quarter them lengthwise and then run them through the slicing blade of a food processor—crosswise, of course.

In a bowl, mix together the vinegar, maple syrup, stevia, and maple extract and pour the mixture over the cukes. Stir it up and chill. When dinnertime rolls around, pull out the salad and season it with salt and pepper.

1½ pounds (680 g) cucumbers

⅓ cup (80 ml) cider vinegar

2 tablespoons (40 g) maple syrup

36 drops of English toffee–flavored liquid stevia extract

3 drops of maple extract

Salt and ground black pepper, to taste

Per serving: 50 calories, trace fat, 1 g protein, 12 g carbohydrate, 1 g dietary fiber, 11 g net carbs

Cucumbers in Mustardy Yogurt Dressing

SERVES 4

Tester Hanftka says, "This is a very simple recipe, with a lot of flavor for not a lot of work and not a lot of carbs. It's a winner."

Scrub the cukes. If they're really big, slice them in half or quarters lengthwise and then run them through the thinnest slicing blade your food processor has—crosswise, of course. Dump 'em in a big mixing bowl.

In a bowl, mix together the yogurt or Coconut Sour Cream and mustard, pour the mixture over the cukes, and stir to coat. Season the mixture with salt and pepper and chill for at least an hour or two before serving.

1½ pounds (680 g) cucumbers

½ cup (115 g) full-fat Greek yogurt, or Coconut Sour Cream (See page 37.)

2 tablespoons (30 g) spicy brown mustard

Salt and ground black pepper, to taste

Per serving: 40 calories, 3 g fat, 2 g protein, 2 g carbohydrate, trace dietary fiber, 2 g net carbs

Jicama Salad

SERVES 6

Crisp, juicy, and mildly sweet, jicama is a beloved part of Mexican cuisine.

Peel the jicama, cut it into chunks that will fit in your food processor, and run it through the shredding blade. Dump this into a nonreactive mixing bowl—stainless steel, glass, or ceramic.

Swap out the shredding blade for the S-blade and mince the onion. Add it to the jicama. Throw in the cilantro, too. Pour the oil on the salad and toss well.

Grate ½ teaspoon lime zest. Roll both limes hard under the heel of your hand before halving and squeezing out the juice into a bowl. Fish out any seeds and then add the juice to the salad and toss well. Season the salad with salt and pepper and chill for at least an hour or two before serving.

1 large jicama

¼ of a large red onion

½ cup (8 g) minced cilantro

⅓ cup (80 ml) avocado oil or light olive oil

2 limes, at room temperature or a little warmer

Salt and ground black pepper, to taste

Per serving 158 calories, 12 g fat, 1 g protein, 13 g carbohydrate, 6 g dietary fiber, 7 g net carbs

Ra-Tato Salad

You are going to be so surprised! Boiling changes radishes entirely; they're mild, with a texture reminiscent of a red-skinned new potato.

Put the radishes in a big saucepan, cover them with water, put the pan over a medium burner, and bring to a simmer. Turn the heat down to medium-low and let them simmer until tender, for about 30 minutes. Drain and let them cool.

Dice the radishes and put them in a mixing bowl. Add the celery and onion. Now add the mayonnaise and stir till everything is evenly coated.

Peel and coarsely chop the eggs. Stir them into the mixture gently, preserving some hunks of yolk. Refrigerate the salad for several hours to let the flavors blend before serving.

1 pound (455 g) radishes, trimmed (See note.)

½ cup (60 g) diced celery

¼ cup (40 g) diced red onion

⅓ cup (75 g) Good Ol' Mayonnaise (See page 30.)

2 eggs, hard-boiled

Per serving: 157 calories, 15 g fat, 3 g protein, 4 g carbohydrate, 2 g dietary fiber, 2 g net carbs

note

The weight for the radishes assumes they're already trimmed. If you buy bunch radishes, with their leaves, you'll need to buy extra to be sure you have enough.

Pineapple-Avocado-Strawberry Fruit Salad

This is very simple, especially if your grocery store sells fresh-cut pineapple chunks. Serve this as a salad or dessert, as you prefer.

In a bowl, gently toss the pineapple, strawberries, and avocado with the dressing. Serve immediately.

1½ cups (233 g) diced pineapple

1½ cups (255 g) quartered strawberries

1 avocado, diced

⅓ cup (80 ml) White Balsamic Vinaigrette (See page 31.)

Per serving: 146 calories, 12 g fat, 1 g protein, 10 g carbohydrate, 2 g dietary fiber, 8 g net carbs

Hot Vegetable Sides

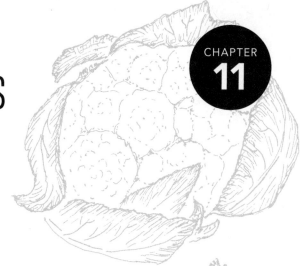

I'm going to take a wild guess that a lot of your meals feature a simple animal protein, such as steaks, chops, burgers, fish fillets, or roasted chicken. They're easy, and they're mostly quick to prepare. But they can also become a little dull day after day.

This is where the hot vegetable side dish comes in. If you put something new and interesting next to that steak or pork chop, you've got a tasty and interesting meal. The fact that vegetables are generally quick-cooking also makes this the swiftest way to add variety to meals.

I'll start with two recipes that will be familiar to those of you who have my previous books. Sorry for the repeat, but they are so useful that they simply must be included.

Caulirice

This is hardly new; it's a staple among low carbers. But it's such a useful idea that I couldn't leave it out. I use this whenever I have chicken in a sauce I'd like to soak up. I also use it in place of rice, orzo, or bulgur in salads of every kind. You'll find a few riffs on Caulirice later in this chapter.

Trim the very bottom of the stem from the half head of cauliflower and trim off the leaves. Whack the remainder into chunks that will fit in your food processor's feed tube. Run it through the shredding blade.

Steam the resulting "caulirice" lightly. (I generally steam mine for 8 minutes on high in my microwave steamer. For the love of all that's holy, don't overcook it. It becomes mushy, and then it's all over.)

SERVES 4

½ of a head of cauliflower

Per serving: 18 calories, trace fat, 1 g protein, 4 g carbohydrate, 2 g dietary fiber, 2 g net carbs

Fauxtatoes

This is another old standard in the low-carb world. Fauxtatoes are a great stand-in for mashed potatoes, especially if you have a super tasty gravy to soak up.

Trim the very bottom of the stem of the half head of cauliflower and remove the leaves. Whack the rest into chunks and steam till tender. (I steamed mine for 12 to 15 minutes on high in my microwave steamer.)

Drain the cauliflower very well. This is vital. Now puree the cauliflower. (I put mine in a deep bowl and use my stick blender. I find the food processor pulverizes it a tad too much.)

Add the sour cream and butter, if using. Mash them in. Season the mashed cauliflower with salt and pepper.

SERVES 3

½ of a head of cauliflower

¼ cup (60 g) sour cream or Coconut Sour Cream, (See page 37.)

2 tablespoons (28 g) butter (optional)

Salt and ground black pepper, to taste

Per serving: 133 calories, 12 g fat, 3 g protein, 6 g carbohydrate, 2 g dietary fiber, 4 g net carbs

Bacon-Walnut Brussels Sprouts

My grocery store has started carrying sliced Brussels sprouts! Hooray! If yours doesn't, your food processor will take care of it in a flash.

Lay the bacon in your biggest skillet over medium heat and fry it until crisp.

Trim the very bottoms of the stems off the Brussels sprouts and remove any wilted leaves. Run them through the slicing blade of your food processor.

Spread the walnuts on a rimmed baking sheet and put 'em in the oven. Turn it to 350°F (180°C or gas mark 4), and set the timer for 12 minutes. (The preheating time is part of the toasting time.) If you're frying the bacon, turn it!

When the bacon is crisp, remove it from the skillet and reserve. Turn the burner up a little to medium-high. Throw in the shallot and sauté it for just a minute or so before adding the Brussels sprouts.

Somewhere in here, your oven timer will beep. Take the walnuts out! You don't want them to burn.

Keep sautéing the Brussels sprouts and shallot, stirring them every minute or two, until the Brussels sprouts have plenty of brown spots. If you need more bacon grease, add a tablespoon or two (14 to 28 g). (I trust you have a bacon grease jar by the stove?)

When the Brussels sprouts are soft and browned, stir in the walnuts and crumble in the bacon. (Actually, I snip mine in with my kitchen shears.) Stir it all up.

3 slices of bacon

12 ounces (340 g) Brussels sprouts, sliced

¼ cup (30 g) chopped walnuts

1 large shallot, minced

1 to 2 tablespoons (14 to 28 g) bacon grease (optional)

Per serving: 109 calories, 7 g fat, 6 g protein, 8 g carbohydrate, 3 g dietary fiber, 5 g net carbs

Maple-Mustard Brussels Sprouts

If you can't get Brussels sprouts sliced, it's quick and easy to run them through the slicing blade of your food processor.

If your sprouts didn't come sliced, do that first, of course. Then put a big, heavy skillet over medium heat. Melt the bacon grease and start sautéing the Brussels sprouts in it, stirring often.

When the Brussels sprouts are turning soft and have plenty of brown spots, stir in the mustard, maple syrup, and water. Keep stirring and cooking for another couple of minutes until the water evaporates. (It's just in there to help the mustard and maple syrup mix into the sprouts better.) Season the Brussels sprouts with salt and pepper.

SERVES 4

12 ounces (340 g) Brussels sprouts, sliced

¼ cup (55 g) bacon grease

1 tablespoon (15 g) spicy brown mustard

1 tablespoon (20 g) maple syrup

1 tablespoon (15 ml) water

Salt and ground black pepper, to taste

Per serving: 168 calories, 14 g fat, 3 g protein, 10 g carbohydrate, 3 g dietary fiber, 7 g net carbs

Bacon Sweetertaters

Even counting the ingredients in the Bacon Jazz, this has still only five, and it's so good you'll serve it for holidays. You can boil or steam the sweet potatoes if you prefer, but baking them concentrates the flavor. See the directions on page 145 to bake 'em in your slow cooker!

Preheat the oven to 350°F (180°C or gas mark 4).

Scrub the sweet potato and rub with a little of the bacon grease. Stick 'er in the oven and let bake until soft. When the tater is soft, pull it out of the oven and let it cool for 15 minutes.

Slice the sweet potato in half and scoop all of the flesh into a mixing bowl. Add the rest of the bacon grease and the Bacon Jazz. Mash it all up and serve immediately!

SERVES 4

1 large sweet potato (1½ pounds, or 680 g)

1 tablespoon (14 g) bacon grease

¼ of the recipe (about 3 tablespoons, or 45 g) for Bacon Jazz (See page 171.)

Per serving: 337 calories, 18 g fat, 11 g protein, 33 g carbohydrate, 4 g dietary fiber, 29 g net carbs

Pink Browns

These are similar to hash browns, only they're pink. If you have a super big skillet, feel free to double this. I just figured everybody had your standard big iron skillet. Or at least they should.

Put a big, heavy skillet over medium heat.

Meanwhile, run the radishes through the shredding blade of your food processor. Run the onion through, too. (I had a couple of bits of onion left that didn't go through the blade. Just mince 'em and throw 'em in.)

Throw the bacon grease in your hot skillet and slosh it around to coat the bottom. Dump in your veggies and spread them into an even layer.

Busy yourself with other things—emptying the dishwasher putting together the rest of the meal. Most of this recipe is waiting for the water to cook out of the radishes. Every 8 to 10 minutes, use a spatula to turn big clumps of the mixture over and spread it out again, letting it cook evenly.

As the water cooks away, your radishes will start to brown. Keep going till the whole thing is well-browned. Season the radishes with salt and pepper.

SERVES 2

1 pound (455 g) radishes, trimmed

⅛ of a medium onion

2 tablespoons (28 g) bacon grease

Salt and ground black pepper, to taste

Per serving: 162 calories, 14 g fat, 1 g protein, 8 g carbohydrate, 3 g dietary fiber, 5 g net carbs

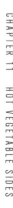

Rutabaga Latkes

SERVES
12

*I am nobody's idea of Jewish, so I can't claim any kind of
authenticity for these. But they're simple, good, and filling.
I also think they're parve (okay to eat with either meat or dairy),
though again, I'm as goyish as they come.*

Preheat the oven to its lowest setting.

Peel the rutabaga half, whack in into chunks, and run it through
the shredding blade of a food processor. Dump the shreds in a
big mixing bowl. Do the same with the onion. If your processor
is like mine, some bits of onion will wind up unshredded. Just
mince them up with a knife and throw them in. Add the eggs
and whisk them in.

In a small bowl, stir together the coconut flour, salt, and pepper.
Now add this to the rutabaga mixture, sprinkling a bit over the
top and whisking, sprinkling then whisking. When it's all in, let
it sit for about 10 minutes.

Heat plenty of oil—⅛ to ¼ inch (3 to 6 mm)—in a big, heavy
skillet. I used an ice cream scoop to make even-sized latkes.
Drop a scoopful in the hot fat and flatten a little, then another.
Fry 'em good and brown before flipping them.

Drain the latkes on paper towels or an old brown paper grocery
sack, and keep them warm in the oven while you finish cooking.

½ of a large rutabaga—about
the size of a grapefruit

1 medium onion

2 eggs

2 tablespoons (14 g) coconut
flour

½ teaspoon salt

¼ teaspoon ground black
pepper

Coconut oil or other fat, to fry

Per serving: 27 calories, 1 g fat,
1 g protein, 3 g carbohydrate,
1 g dietary fiber, 2 g net carbs

notes

We ate these as-is, as a side dish, but you can add a little sour cream or
Coconut Sour Cream (see page 37) if you like.

Don't skimp on the oil! Latkes are traditional for Hanukah, when oily foods
are eaten in commemoration of the oil lighting the temple lasting 8 days.

It would be as inauthentic as it gets, but these would be quite tasty fried in
bacon grease. If you do this, call them Rutabaga Fritters.

Broccoli with Olives and Pine Nuts

SERVES
6

This preparation plays up broccoli's Mediterranean heritage. I used a combination of Kalamata olives and green olives packed in olive oil, with a few hot peppers in the mix. Just be sure to use good, strong-flavored olives.

Start by cutting the stems off the broccoli, not to discard them, but to make them easier to peel. Use a paring knife to peel the tough skin from the stems and then cut them into bite-sized pieces. (If you've never done this before, you may be startled to discover the stems are the best part!) Cut up the florets into similar-sized bites, again, peeling any tough skin. Set this to steam. (I steamed mine for 10 minutes in the microwave, but do yours on the stovetop, if you prefer.)

While the broccoli is steaming, stir the pine nuts in a medium-sized dry skillet over medium heat until they're golden.

Okay, the ten minutes are up. Check the broccoli for doneness. (You want it tender but not mushy.) If it needs another minute or two, do that. Otherwise, uncover it.

In the meantime, remove the pine nuts from the skillet to a small plate and keep them close at hand. Turn the burner back on under the skillet, this time to medium-low, and add the butter. Let it melt and then stir in the lemon juice and the olives.

Put the broccoli in a big bowl and pour the butter-lemon-olive mixture over it. Toss the mixture to coat thoroughly. Sprinkle the pine nuts over the top and toss it again.

2 pounds (900 g) broccoli

¼ cup (34 g) pine nuts

¼ cup (55 g) butter

¼ cup (25 g) chopped Kalamata olives, green olives, or a combo

2 tablespoons (28 ml) lemon juice

Per serving: 135 calories, 12 g fat, 4 g protein, 6 g carbohydrate, 3 g dietary fiber, 3 g net carbs

Cauliflower with Bacon

As we all know, bacon improves everything it touches. This cauliflower is simple and amazing. Don't be surprised if the kids are fighting over the last few bits.

Preheat the oven to 450°F (230°C or gas mark 8). While it's heating, put the bacon grease in a dark metal roasting pan and slide it in the oven to melt.

Chop the cauliflower into bite-sized chunks. Snip or chop the bacon into little bits.

Pull the melted bacon grease out of the oven. Throw in the cauliflower and bacon and toss till everything is intimately acquainted. Put the whole thing back in the oven and roast it for 5 minutes.

When the timer beeps, use a spatula to stir and turn everything over. Keep roasting, stirring and turning every 5 minutes, until the bacon is crisp and the cauliflower is well browned. Serve immediately.

SERVES 3

2 tablespoons (28 g) bacon grease

½ of a head of cauliflower

2 slices of bacon

Per serving: 107 calories, 11 g fat, 2 g protein, 1 g carbohydrate, trace dietary fiber, 1 g net carbs

Creamed Spinach

That Nice Boy I Married, a true spinach lover, yummed this right down, and he would have eaten more. You could try to double this, but geez, you'd need a big skillet.

Put a big, heavy skillet over low heat. Add the coconut oil and let it melt. Now add the garlic and the anchovies. Sauté them together, breaking up the anchovies with your spatula till the anchovies have pretty much dissolved. Now throw in the spinach. Sauté, turning the mass over from time to time, just until it has all softened and deflated. Stir in the coconut milk and let it heat through. Season the spinach with salt and pepper.

SERVES 3

2 tablespoons (24 g) coconut oil

1 clove of garlic, crushed

2 anchovy fillets

10 ounces (280 g) fresh spinach

½ cup (120 ml) coconut milk

Salt and ground black pepper, to taste

Per serving: 198 calories, 19 g fat, 4 g protein, 6 g carbohydrate, 3 g dietary fiber, 3 g net carbs

Easy Cookout Mushrooms

SERVES
3

If it's snowing outside or you don't feel like grilling, you could bake these in the oven for around 45 minutes at 350°F (180°C or gas mark 4). I'd put them in a roasting pan in case the packet springs a leak.

Tear off a big piece of heavy-duty foil and lay it on the counter. If you're using oil instead of butter, bend the edges up a bit.

Put the mushrooms in the center of the foil. Scatter the garlic over them. Dot with the butter or drizzle with the oil. Scatter the parsley over that. Lightly season the mushrooms with salt and pepper.

Bring the ends of the foil up over the mushrooms and roll down. Now roll in the ends, making a tight packet. Throw the packet on the grill. Let it cook for about 15 to 20 minutes, turning it from time to time with tongs. (The timing will depend on how hot the fire is.)

When it's done, open the packet on a plate and serve with a spoon. There will be plenty of flavorful juice inside.

½ pound (225 g) mushrooms

1 clove of garlic, crushed

3 tablespoons (42 g) butter or (45 ml) olive oil

1 tablespoon (4 g) minced fresh parsley

Salt and ground black pepper, to taste

Per serving: 122 calories, 12 g fat, 2 g protein, 4 g carbohydrate, 1 g dietary fiber, 3 g net carbs

Savory Mushrooms

SERVES
2

Don't be afraid of anchovies. I'm not a fan of anchovies by themselves, but here they just add savor. If you're really nervous, back it off to two anchovies the first time. Serve this over steak or use it as an omelet filling.

Put a big, heavy skillet over medium-high heat. Pour in the oil and add the anchovies. Mash 'em with a fork till they kind of dissolve into the oil. Add the mushrooms and garlic and sauté until the mushrooms are soft. Stir in the parsley and serve immediately.

¼ cup (60 ml) olive oil

3 anchovy fillets

8 ounces (225 g) sliced mushrooms

2 cloves of garlic, crushed

¼ cup (15 g) minced fresh parsley

Per serving: 143 calories, 14 g fat, 2 g protein, 3 g carbohydrate, 1 g dietary fiber, 2 g net carbs

Garlicky Mushrooms with Sun-Dried Tomatoes

SERVES
4

8 ounces (225 g) sliced mushrooms

3 tablespoons (45 ml) olive oil

¼ cup (28 g) sun-dried tomatoes in olive oil, chopped fine

4 cloves of garlic, crushed

Per serving: 123 calories, 11 g fat, 2 g protein, 5 g carbohydrate, 1 g dietary fiber, 4 g net carbs

Do you need something to dress up a simple hamburger patty or chicken breast? These are perfect. Have someone to impress? Serve them over steak. Making brunch? These are a perfect omelet filling. You can't go wrong!

Put your big, heavy skillet over medium-low heat and start the mushrooms sautéing in the oil. Add 1 tablespoon (15 ml) of oil from the sun-dried tomato jar to the mushrooms for extra flavor.

When the mushrooms are getting soft, add the tomatoes. Sauté them for another couple of minutes and then stir in the garlic. Give them another minute or two and then serve or stash them in the fridge as a quick way to dress up a meal.

Easy Sweet Potato Wedges

SERVES
6

⅓ cup (85 g) bacon grease

2 sweet potatoes

Creole Seasoning (See page 35.)

Per serving: 151 calories, 12 g fat, 1 g protein, 11 g carbohydrate, 1 g dietary fiber, 10 g net carbs

Cutting up the sweet potatoes reduces the baking time by a good 30 minutes.

Preheat the oven to 375°F (190°C or gas mark 5). Put the bacon grease in a big roasting pan and slide it into the oven to melt.

Scrub the sweet potatoes well. Now half them lengthwise and then cut them into slices about ½ inch (1.3 cm) thick.

Pull the pan out of the oven. Throw in the sweet potato bits and use a spatula to stir and turn them till they're coated with bacon grease. Sprinkle them well with the Creole Seasoning.

Bake the potatoes for 15 minutes. Pull them out of the oven, use your spatula to flip them all, and then sprinkle the other side with Creole Seasoning, too. Bake the potatoes for another 15 minutes and then serve.

Totally Inauthentic Dirty "Rice"

This recipe assumes you've made the Savory Roast Chicken on page 65, but that's not essential. Any time you roast a chicken, you can use the giblets this way. This is one of the most complex dishes in the book; I offer it as a way to get organ meats into your diet. I consider all the chicken detritus—the giblets, their broth and the drippings in the roasting pan—as one ingredient.

Put the neck, heart, and gizzard in a small saucepan, cover with water, and bring to a simmer. Let them simmer until tender. Drop the liver into the giblet pan, cover, and remove from heat. (You're letting the residual heat gently poach the liver.)

Put the chicken giblets in a roasting pan and keep them warm. (Your oven set to its very lowest heat works well for this.)

Cut the celery and onion into chunks and drop 'em in your food processor. Pulse till they're chopped medium-fine.

Put a big, heavy skillet over medium heat. Add the fat, celery, and onions and start them sautéing.

Put the food processor bowl back on the base and swap out the S-blade for the shredding blade. Chunk the cauliflower, including the stem, and run it through the shredding blade.

Go stir the celery and onions. Are they getting a little soft? Good. Throw in the cauliflower and mix it all together.

Pour the broth off the giblets into the pan you roasted the chicken in and stir, scraping up all the nice brown stuff, dissolving it into the broth. Pour this into the cauliflower mixture and again, stir. (If you didn't roast a chicken prior to making this recipe, simply pour the broth directly into the cauliflower mixture.) Bring to a simmer. Let it cook while you dice the giblets fine, including any meat you can pick off the neck. (Skip the skin. It'll be gooey.)

When the Caulirice is tender and the broth has mostly cooked down, stir in the giblets and the Creole Seasoning. You're done!

---

1 set of chicken giblets

1 large rib of celery

1 small onion

3 tablespoons (42 g) chicken fat, lard, or bacon grease

½ of a head of cauliflower

1 tablespoon (11 g) Creole Seasoning (See page 35.)

Per serving: 145 calories, 11 g fat, 6 g protein, 7 g carbohydrate, 2 g dietary fiber, 5 g net carbs

Green Goddess "Rice"

*This is unusual, creamy, and good! Try it with chicken or fish.
You could stir cooked shrimp into this to make a one-dish meal,
and you'd still be under five ingredients!*

Trim the leaves and the very bottom of the stem of the half head
of cauliflower and then whack it into chunks and run it through
the shredding blade of your food processor. Steam it till barely
tender. (I steamed mine for 8 minutes on high in my microwave
steamer, but do it on the stovetop if you prefer.)

While the cauliflower is steaming, scoop the avocado flesh
out of the skin into a bowl. Add the pesto and mash the whole
thing with a fork until you have a creamy sauce with a scattering
of chunks of avocado. Or you can put the avocado and pesto
in a food processor and pulse.

When the cauliflower is done, drain off any excess water and
stir in the sauce. Season with salt.

SERVES 4

½ of a head of cauliflower

1 avocado, pitted

¼ cup (65 g) pesto sauce

Salt, to taste

Per serving: 175 calories, 15 g fat,
5 g protein, 9 g carbohydrate,
3 g dietary fiber, 6 g net carbs

note

With the addition of 1½ to 2 cups
(210 to 280 g) of diced leftover
chicken or turkey, this becomes
a great one dish meal.

Maple-Chipotle Pumpkin

*It's a shame sugar pumpkins—the little ones—are only available
in the autumn. They're good for much more than pie.*

Whack the pumpkin in half and scoop out the seeds, saving
them for Dirty Punks (see page 39).

Put a small saucepan over low heat and melt the butter into the
maple syrup. Stir in the hot sauce.

Grill the pumpkin over well ashed charcoal. When it's getting soft,
start basting it with the maple mixture every 5 minutes or so, until
it's good and soft. Serve the pumpkin with a little more glaze
spooned over it. (You can also roast the pumpkin wedges in the
oven. Again, start glazing them when they start getting soft.)

SERVES 8

2 pounds (900 g) sugar pumpkin

¼ cup (55 g) butter

½ cup (160 g) maple syrup

1 tablespoon (15 ml) chipotle
hot sauce

Per serving: 132 calories, 6 g fat,
1 g protein, 21 g carbohydrate,
1 g dietary fiber, 20 g net carbs

Slow Cooker Acorn Squash

SERVES 2

This worked beautifully! No more baking squash for an hour. It can be ready when you get home. And with this seasoning, it could serve as dessert.

Whack the squash in half and scoop out the innards. Save the seeds for Dirty Punks (see page 39).

In a small saucepan, melt the butter and mix in the pumpkin pie spice and stevia.

Put one half of the squash in a slow cooker and spoon a little less than half of the butter mixture into it. Use a basting brush to spread a little more of the mixture on the cut sides.

Settle the second squash half down on the first. (This is the only way to fit the halves in my 4 quart [3.8 L] slow cooker, and if you cut the bits smaller, you lose that nice hollow.) Spoon more butter-spice mixture into the second half and spread the last of it on the cut sides. Cover the slow cooker and set to high. Let it cook for 5 to 6 hours.

Use a big, big spoon to lift out the squash halves and place them on plates to serve.

1 acorn squash

¼ cup (55 g) butter

½ teaspoon pumpkin pie spice

Scant ¼ teaspoon English toffee–flavored liquid stevia extract

Per serving: 291 calories, 23 g fat, 2 g protein, 23 g carbohydrate, 3 g dietary fiber, 20 g net carbs

Vermouth-Braised Fennel

Elegant and unusual, this fennel dish is fit for a holiday or company. Try it with a simple fish dish and a salad.

Preheat the oven to 350°F (180°C or gas mark 4).

Whack the stems off of the fennel bulbs and trim the very bottoms. Now cut them each lengthwise into 8 wedges.

Put an ovenproof skillet over medium heat. When it's hot, add the oil and then the fennel. Season the fennel with salt and pepper a bit as it sautés. (You want to just brown it on either flat side of each wedge.)

In a bowl, stir together the vermouth and broth and pour the mixture over the fennel. Cover the skillet and stick the whole thing in the oven. Let it cook for 20 minutes or until soft. Serve the fennel with the pan juices poured over it.

4 bulbs of fennel

¼ cup (60 ml) olive oil

Salt and ground black pepper, to taste

½ cup (120 ml) dry vermouth

1 cup (235 ml) chicken broth

Per serving: 236 calories, 14 g fat, 4 g protein, 19 g carbohydrate, 7 g dietary fiber, 12 g net carbs

note

If you don't have an oven-safe skillet, you can transfer the sautéed fennel to a baking dish to finish. If you have an oven-safe skillet, but not an oven-safe lid —hey, that's what foil is for.

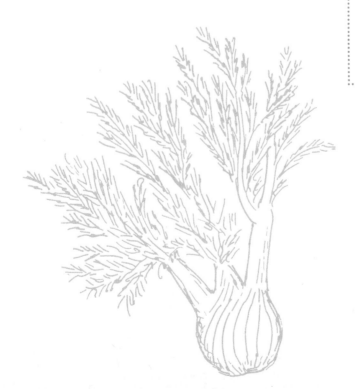

Almond Butter Green Beans

SERVES
4

I saw a recipe called Green Beans with Almond Butter, and I thought, "Interesting!" It turned out to just be good old Green Beans Almondine. But the idea stuck with me, and I came up with this.

Trim the green beans and cut them in shorter lengths or leave whole, as you prefer. Steam them till just tender. (I steamed mine for 10 minutes in the microwave steamer, but use the stovetop if you prefer.)

In the meantime, put a small saucepan over low heat and melt the butter and almond butter together. Stir in the lemon juice.

When the beans are just tender, drain 'em and toss them with the sauce till coated, season with salt, and then serve immediately.

1 pound (455 g) green beans

2 tablespoons (28 g) butter

3 tablespoons (45 g) almond butter

1½ tablespoons (25 ml) lemon juice

Salt, to taste

Per serving: 154 calories, 12 g fat, 4 g protein, 10 g carbohydrate, 5 g dietary fiber, 5 g net carbs

Savory Green Beans

SERVES
4

If you'd like to speed this up, you could use frozen green beans. Just read the label to make sure that nothing has been added to them.

Snip the ends off of the green beans and then cut them into 1½- to 2-inch (3.8 to 5 cm) lengths. (I use my kitchen shears for this.) Either in the microwave or on the stovetop, steam the beans until tender. (I steamed mine for 10 minutes in my microwave steamer.)

In the meantime, put a big skillet over medium heat and use kitchen shears to snip the bacon into it. Let it start frying out into nice little bacon bits. When the bacon bits are about half done, add the shallot to the skillet and stir it in.

Keep sautéing until the bacon bits are crisp and the shallot has browned. Stir in the green beans, tossing till everything is well blended. Season the beans with salt and pepper.

1½ pounds (680 g) green beans

3 slices of bacon

1 shallot, minced

Salt and ground black pepper, to taste

Per serving: 76 calories, 2 g fat, 4 g protein, 11 g carbohydrate, 5 g dietary fiber, 6 g net carbs

Green Bean and Pepper Sauté

This is easy and delicious, and it also looks beautiful on the plate. You could make it even prettier by using red onion, though I think the stronger flavor of yellow onions is good here. You could use frozen beans here if you wanted to. Look for whole frozen beans for the spiffiest looking presentation.

Trim the green beans.

Put a big, heavy skillet over medium low heat and add the pine nuts. Stir till they're golden. Remove to a plate and reserve.

Put the skillet back over the burner and turn the heat up to medium high. Melt half of the butter or oil and throw in the green beans. Stir them around to coat and then cover the skillet. Cook the beans for 5 minutes.

In the meantime, cut the pepper through the equator, then in half lengthwise, and then into strips a little narrower than the green beans.

The timer beeped! Stir the beans, re-cover the skillet, and cook the beans for another 5 minutes. There's that beep again. Stir the beans and check for doneness. (The timing will depend on how fresh they are.) When the beans are still a bit al dente, melt in the rest of the butter or oil, and then add the pepper and onion. Stir it up! Re-cover the skillet and cook the mixture for another 5 minutes. Serve the beans, onion, and peppers topped with the pine nuts.

1 pound (455 g) green beans

¼ cup (35 g) pine nuts

¼ cup (53 g) butter or (60 ml) olive oil, divided (The butter adds a lot.)

1 large yellow bell pepper

2 tablespoons (20 g) minced onion

Per serving: 89 calories, 5 g fat, 4 g protein, 11 g carbohydrate, 4 g dietary fiber, 7 g net carbs

Lemon-Garlic Green Beans

You can do this with just olive oil if you prefer, but I think the butter–olive oil combo is awfully good.

Snip the ends off of the green beans. Put your biggest skillet over medium-high heat. Add the butter and oil and swirl them together as the butter melts. Throw in the beans. Sauté them, stirring every minute or so, until they're turning bright green. Stir in the garlic and grate in the zest from the lemon half. (It's easier to grate it from the lemon while it's whole, and then cut it in half to get juice.) Keep stirring the beans every minute or two.

When the beans are tender, squeeze in the juice from the lemon half, and stir it in. Let the beans cook just for another minute and then serve immediately.

1½ pounds (680 g) green beans

2 tablespoons (28 g) butter

2 tablespoons (28 ml) olive oil

2 cloves of garlic, crushed

½ of a lemon

Per serving: 107 calories, 8 g fat, 2 g protein, 8 g carbohydrate, 3 g dietary fiber, 5 g net carbs

Turnips with Mushrooms and Shallots

Peasant food of legend, turnips get a major upgrade with this treatment. Top any leftovers with fried eggs for breakfast.

Cut the turnips in a ½-inch (1.3 cm) dice or use your food processor to chop them to chunks roughly that size. Put them in a steamer and steam for 8 minutes.

Chop the mushrooms and peel and mince the shallot.

Put a big, heavy skillet over medium-low heat and melt the butter. Start sautéing the mushrooms and shallot, stirring now and then. When the turnips are done, drain off any excess water and then add them to the skillet and stir them in. Turn the burner up a little to just below medium. Cook, turning everything over now and then, until the turnips brown. Serve immediately.

3 medium turnips—about tennis ball–sized, peeled

4 ounces (115 g) mushrooms

1 shallot

¼ cup (55 g) butter

Per serving: 135 calories, 12 g fat, 2 g protein, 7 g carbohydrate, 2 g dietary fiber, 5 g net carbs

Slow Cooker Caramelized Onions

SERVES
12

Caramelized onions improve so many things. But knowing that they take 20 to 25 minutes can put you off, especially if the family is howling for dinner now! *Make a slow cooker full, stash them in the freezer, and you'll have them at your fingertips.*

¼ cup (55 g) lard, bacon grease, coconut oil, or (60 ml) olive oil

6 onions

Per serving: 59 calories, 4 g fat, 1 g protein, 5 g carbohydrate, 1 g dietary fiber, 4 g nets carbs

Put the fat in a small saucepan and set it over a low burner to melt.

Whack the onions in half, peel them, cut off the ends, and run them through the slicing blade of your food processor. (You didn't think I was going to make you cry that hard, did you?)

Dump the onions into the slow cooker. Drizzle the melted fat over them as you stir them a bit with a big spoon. (You want to coat them as evenly as you can.)

Cover the slow cooker, set it on low, and let it go for 8 hours or so.

Voilà! You now are the proud possessor of a big stash of caramelized onions! Divide them up into batches that will work for your life, depending on how many people you're feeding, package 'em up (I put mine in zipper-lock sandwich bags) and throw them in the freezer. Haul them out whenever you want something special on a steak, a burger, a chop, or whatever.

note

Six medium onions are about what will fit in your average 4-quart (3.8 L) slow cooker. You can use more or fewer if you've got a bigger one or a smaller one. Really, just fill your slow cooker with sliced onions, pour in some melted fat, stir, cover, and cook on low till they're golden.

Slow Cooker Baked Sweet Potatoes

If you eat sweet potatoes often, you may as well cook extra. Serve them with butter or anything else you like. The next day, slice them and fry them brown in bacon grease.

Wrap each sweet potato tightly in foil. Put them in a slow cooker, stacking them if need be.

Cover your slow cooker, set it to low, and go to work. Let them cook for 8 hours or so. (You'll come home to a house full of the sweet smell of baked sweets.)

SERVES 8

4 large sweet potatoes, scrubbed

Per serving: 68 calories, trace fat, 1 g protein, 16 g carbohydrate, 2 g dietary fiber, 14 g net carbs

Slow Cooker Beets

Come home to roasted beets for dinner. You can simply slice or dice and butter them or use them in salads, such as the Beet and Orange Salad on page 123.

Trim the leaves off of the beets, leaving the stem and root ends intact. (This keeps the juice in.) Scrub them well and dry them.

Tear off 6 squares of foil, each big enough for a beet. In turn, lay each beet on a square of foil, and give it a nice massage with a teaspoon of the fat. Wrap it up into a nice tight bundle and drop it in your slow cooker. Repeat until all the beets are in the slow cooker.

Cover the slow cooker, set it to low, and go have a life for 8 hours. When you come back, squeeze the biggest of your beets gently, using an oven mitt, of course. If it's soft, they're done. If not, have a glass of wine and give them another hour or so.

When the beets are done, run them under cold water and rub off the skins. Trim the stem and root ends. Serve.

SERVES 8

6 medium beets

2 tablespoons (28 g) fat of your choice

Per serving: 56 calories, 4 g fat, 1 g protein, 6 g carbohydrate, 2 g dietary fiber, 4 g net carbs

Soups

In my kitchen freezer there lives two plastic grocery sacks. One houses the bones of all the chicken we eat, the other any beef bones we manage to accumulate. I throw in onion and celery trimmings—going easy on celery leaves, which can be bitter—and maybe a carrot top or two.

When a sack becomes full enough to mess with closing the freezer drawer, I dump the contents into my stockpot or my biggest slow cooker, cover with water, and a teaspoon of salt and a glug of apple cider or wine vinegar—maybe ¼ cup (60 ml). I set the stockpot over my simmer burner, or turn the slow cooker to low, and let it cook for 24 hours or so. What's the result? It's bone broth, also known as pure nutritional magic. You owe it to yourself to buy meat on the bone, if only to accumulate bones for broth.

I know lots of people who simply drink a cup or two (235 to 475 ml) of bone broth per day, and that's a fine idea. But if you'd like something a little more interesting, here you go.

You can cheat with good boxed stock. Dissolve a couple of tablespoons (14 g) of unflavored gelatin in it to give it the body it lacks. I also have been known to boil boxed stock hard to reduce by about a third to intensify the flavor. But good bone broth is so seriously worth the very little time and money it takes.

Turkey Min-Not-Strone

SERVES
8

This is the perfect soup for the Sunday after Thanksgiving! This has to be started the day before because you need to boil up the turkey carcass, but there's nothing hard here or that takes a lot of work.

Put the turkey carcass in a big stockpot and cover it with water. If there are any herbs, onions, lemons, or other foods in the cavity, go ahead and include them. Add the salt and bring to a very low simmer. If your carcass is too big to completely submerge in the pot (mine was), let it simmer for 4 to 5 hours and then break it up a bit to get it all under the water. Let it cook for a minimum of 18 hours, and 24 hours isn't too long. Let it cool.

Strain the broth and put it back in the pot. Bring it back to a simmer and let it cook down to about 2 quarts (1.8 L). (This concentrates the flavor.)

In the meantime, pick the meat off of the bones. Cut it into bite-sized pieces and stash it in the fridge till the broth has cooked down. Toss the bones.

Okay, your broth has reduced. Stir in the marinara sauce and the green beans.

Quarter your zukes lengthwise and then slice 'em about ¼ inch (6 mm) thick. Dice the onion.

Put a big, heavy skillet over medium heat and add the oil. Sauté the zucchini and onion until the onion is translucent. Add this all to the soup. Let the whole thing simmer till the green beans are soft. Stir in the turkey bits and bring it back to a simmer.

1 turkey carcass

1 teaspoon salt

1 jar (25 ounces, or 710 g) marinara sauce

1 pound (455 g) green beans, cut into 1½-inch (3.8 cm) lengths (I used frozen, but use fresh if you prefer.)

2 small zucchini, about 7 inches (18 cm) long

1 large onion

¼ cup (60 ml) olive oil

Per serving: 259 calories, 14 g fat, 20 g protein, 14 g carbohydrate, 4 g dietary fiber, 10 g net carbs

note

This nutrition analysis is approximate because I have no way of knowing how big your carcass is, nor how much meat is left on it. If you're eating primal, a sprinkle of grated Parmesan is good on this.

Egg Drop Soup

Like all soups, this is best when made with good, strong, homemade bone broth. But you can cheat, if you like, and use boxed organic chicken stock. I've done it with Kirkland Brand, from Costco. This is especially useful if you're home sick. You might want to dissolve a tablespoon (7 g) or so of unflavored gelatin powder in the boxed stock to give it some of the body it lacks—and more nutritional value, too.

It's so simple! In a saucepan, combine the broth and the Basic Stir-Fry Sauce. Bring the mixture to a simmer.

In the meantime, break the eggs into a glass measuring cup and beat them with a fork, mixing them till there are no big globs of white.

When the broth reaches a simmer, turn the burner down just a little, so it's just below a simmer. Pour in the eggs, a bit at a time, while stirring slowly with a fork. When all the egg is worked in, add the scallions and serve!

SERVES 3

1 quart (950 ml) chicken broth

¼ cup (60 ml) Basic Stir-Fry Sauce (See page 33.)

2 eggs

2 scallions, thinly sliced (optional)

Per serving: 121 calories, 5 g fat, 10 g protein, 5 g carbohydrate, trace dietary fiber, 5 g net carbs

Exotic Pumpkin Soup

I got the idea for this when I bought some wonderful ras el hanout—*a Moroccan spice blend similar to curry—at Sahara Mart, my local international market. I had a can of pumpkin to use up and the rest just happened.*

In a big, heavy-bottomed saucepan over medium-low heat, melt the butter. Add the garlic and *ras el hanout* and sauté them, stirring often, for just a couple of minutes.

Add everything else, stir it up, and bring to a simmer. Let it cook for 15 minutes or so, just to blend the flavors, and then serve.

SERVES 5

2 tablespoons (28 g) butter

3 cloves of garlic, crushed

2 tablespoons (12 g) *ras el hanout*

1 quart (950 ml) chicken broth

1 can (15 ounces, or 425 g) pumpkin

1 can (14 ounces, or 390 ml) unsweetened coconut milk

Per serving: 229 calories, 22 g fat, 6 g protein, 5 g carbohydrate, trace dietary fiber, 5 g net carbs

Immediate Curried Cream of Chicken Soup

My freezer was full of chicken bones, so I made a pot of broth. Because I was working on a cookbook and all, I had to come up with something to do with it immediately. Hence the name.

In a big, heavy saucepan over medium heat, melt the butter and cook the curry powder for just a minute or two.

Add the broth, salsa, and coconut milk. Turn up the burner a bit, so it comes to a simmer.

While the soup is heating, cut your chicken thighs into a dice. (I made mine somewhere between ¼ and ½ inch [0.6 and 1.3 cm]).

Stir the chicken into the soup and let the whole thing simmer for 10 minutes till the chicken cubes are cooked. Season the soup with salt and serve immediately.

SERVES 4

2 tablespoons (28 g) butter

2 tablespoons (13 g) curry powder

1 quart (950 ml) chicken broth

1 jar (16 ounces, or 455 g) + 1 cup (260 g) salsa

14 ounces (390 ml) unsweetened coconut milk

3 boneless, skinless chicken thighs

Salt, to taste

Per serving: 391 calories, 31 g fat, 15 g protein, 16 g carbohydrate, 4 g dietary fiber, 12 g net carbs

Clam Bisque

This soup is creamy, warm, and filling. But read the labels on the clams. I have no idea what possesses people to put sugar in clams, but some companies do.

Put a big, heavy saucepan over low heat and use kitchen shears to snip the bacon into it. Fry the bacon bits till crispy. Scoop them out with a slotted spoon, leaving the grease. Put the bacon bits on a plate and reserve.

Throw the onion and celery into the bacon grease and sauté them till they're softened. Add the water and bring the mixture to a simmer. Cover the pan, turn the burner quite low, and let it simmer for 10 to 15 minutes.

Now stir in the coconut milk and clams, juice and all. Bring the mixture back to a simmer. Serve the soup topped with the bacon.

SERVES 3

2 slices of bacon

¼ cup (40 g) minced onion

¼ cup (30 g) minced celery

¾ cup (175 ml) water

1 can (14 ounces, or 390 ml) unsweetened coconut milk

13 ounces (365 g) canned chopped clams

Per serving: 446 calories, 30 g fat, 34 g protein, 11 g carbohydrate, trace dietary fiber, 11 g net carbs

Streamlined Sopa Azteca

SERVES
3

A favorite among my recipes is Sopa Azteca, a Mexican-style chicken-vegetable soup. It has considerably more than five ingredients! This version can be put together in no time flat.

In your big, nonreactive pot—stainless steel, enamel, or nonstick hard-anodized aluminum—over medium-high heat, combine the broth and salsa. Bring the mixture to a simmer.

This is a good time to dice up the chicken or turkey. One of the joys of this recipe is that it doesn't matter if it's leftover cooked chicken or turkey or if you're starting with boneless, skinless breast, thighs, or turkey cutlets. It's all good. Dice it up. Stir the chicken into the broth-and-salsa mixture. If you're using raw poultry, stir for 30 seconds or so to keep it from congealing into a lump at the bottom of the pot.

That's it for the cooking part. When the time comes to serve the soup, peel, pit and dice the avocado and shred the cheese if you're using it. (Only dice as much avocado and shred as much cheese as you're going to use immediately.)

If you're using the cheese, put a handful in the bottom of each bowl. Ladle hot soup over it, top with chunks of avocado, and serve immediately.

2 quarts (1.9 L) chicken or turkey broth

24 ounces (680 g) chipotle salsa

3 cups (420 g) diced chicken or turkey (This can be leftover cooked chicken or turkey or raw boneless skinless breast or thighs or turkey cutlets.)

3 avocados

1½ cups (170 g) shredded queso quesadilla cheese or (173 g) Monterey Jack cheese (optional)

Per serving: 594 calories, 43 g fat, 37 g protein, 17 g carbohydrate, 4 g dietary fiber, 13 g net carbs

note

This is so quick and simple, it can be thrown together in 15 minutes or so if you have the ingredients on hand. This not only makes it a great weeknight supper, but it's also a terrific choice when you've got a bad cold.

Italian Cream of Chicken Soup

SERVES 8

So I'm looking at this recipe for a chicken dish with sun-dried tomatoes and onions and cream and a bunch of seasonings, and I thought, "That'll never make the five-ingredient limit." But then I thought, "I can make it a soup!" So I did. And it's lovely. If you're eating primal instead of Paleo, a sprinkle of grated Parmesan is good on this, but it's far from essential.

In a big saucepan, combine the broth, marinara sauce, coconut milk, and anchovies. Bring the mixture to a simmer.

Stir in the chicken. Season the soup with salt, and add about ½ teaspoon pepper. (The quantity of salt and pepper will depend upon your broth and your sauce.) Let it simmer for 10 minutes or so and serve immediately.

1 quart (950 ml) chicken broth

1 jar (24 ounces, or 680 g) marinara sauce

1 can (14 ounces, or 390 ml) unsweetened coconut milk

4 anchovies, mashed

3 cups (420 g) diced chicken

Salt, to taste

½ teaspoon ground black pepper, plus more, to taste

Per serving: 474 calories, 35 g fat, 28 g protein, 12 g carbohydrate, 2 g dietary fiber, 10 g net carbs

notes

The nutrition evaluation will vary a bit with your brand of marinara sauce. You can make this with leftover chicken, as I did, or you can dice up boneless, skinless breasts, thighs, or both. If you use raw chicken, stir it into the simmering soup and keep stirring for 20 to 30 seconds. If you just dump it in, it will congeal into a lump in the bottom of your pan, and you'll have to break it apart later.

This is actually very good without the chicken, as a starter, and of course, it's dead simple. For that matter, it would be good with spinach in it instead of, or in addition to, the chicken. A bag of baby spinach would work, or a 10-ounce (280 g) box of frozen, chopped spinach. Zucchini would be good in here, too. Play with it.

CHAPTER 12 SOUPS

151

Main Dish Salads

I love main dish salads! I confess, however, to a general urge to throw a lot of ingredients into them. These, I am pleased to say, are glorious in their simplicity. And remember: If you have cooked protein—leftover steak or chicken, a handful of shrimp, or whatever—some bagged greens, and salad dressing on hand, you are never more than 5 minutes away from a good meal.

Chicken Salad with Grapes

SERVES 3

Simple and classic, this chicken salad is a long-time favorite. Grapes are one of those fruits that make the "Dirty Dozen" list (see page 14). Pop for the organic ones, okay?

Cut all the stuff up—I used the end of a roasted chicken—and throw it in a mixing bowl. Add the mayo and stir to coat. Season the salad with salt and pepper.

2 cups (280 g) diced cooked chicken

½ cup (50 g) chopped celery

4 scallions, sliced

24 red seedless grapes, halved

⅓ cup (75 g) Good Ol' Mayonnaise (See page 30.)

Salt and ground black pepper, to taste

Per serving: 371 calories, 25 g fat, 30 g protein, 9 g carbohydrate, 1 g dietary fiber, 9 g net carbs

Chicken, Avocado, and Bacon Salad

SERVES 3

Oh, c'mon. Just reading that title, you know you want to make this. It's three of the most perfect foods on earth together! If you've got some lettuce on hand, this makes nice lettuce wraps.

Cook the bacon until crisp by whatever method you favor.

In the meantime, cube the chicken and avocado and slice the scallions, including the crisp part of the green. Throw 'em all in a mixing bowl.

Add the Honey Mustard Dressing and stir it all up. Serve with the bacon crumbled on top.

3 slices of bacon

1½ cups (210 g) cooked chicken

1 avocado

2 scallions

¼ cup (60 ml) Honey Mustard Dressing and Dipping Sauce (See page 33.)

Per serving: 387 calories, 29 g fat, 26 g protein, 8 g carbohydrate, 2 g dietary fiber, 6 g net carbs

Chicken (or Turkey) Divan Salad

SERVES
4

I'm a huge fan of Chicken or Turkey Divan, so the idea of the same flavors in a salad struck me as awesome. I was right.

Steam the broccoli. (I gave mine 8 minutes in the microwave, but do yours on the stovetop if you prefer. You want it brilliantly green and tender-crisp.)

In the meantime, place the chicken or turkey in a big bowl.

When the broccoli is done, uncover it immediately to stop the cooking, or you'll end up with a nasty, gray, sulfurous mush. Let it cool for a few minutes.

In a bowl, stir the mayonnaise and vermouth together.

When the broccoli is just warm, add it to the chicken or turkey. Pour on the mayo mixture and stir to coat. Stir in half of the cheese. Serve the salad and sprinkle 1 tablespoon (5 g) of the remaining cheese over each serving.

3 cups (213 g) broccoli, cut into bite-sized bits

2 cups (280 g) diced cooked chicken or turkey

¾ cup (175 g) Good Ol' Mayonnaise (See page 30.)

2 tablespoons (28 ml) vermouth

½ cup (40 g) shredded Parmesan or (50 g) Romano cheese, divided

Per serving: 607 calories, 55 g fat, 27 g protein, 4 g carbohydrate, 2 g dietary fiber, 2 g net carbs

Chicken (or Turkey) Salad Piccata

SERVES
2

This dish offers flavors as bright and warm as the Mediterranean sun. Some parsley would be nice here, if you have the patience to cut up one more ingredient.

This is pretty self-explanatory: Place the chicken or turkey, scallions, and capers in a bowl. Add the mayonnaise and lemon and stir to coat. That's it!

1 cup (140 g) diced cooked chicken or turkey

¼ cup (25 g) thinly sliced scallions

2 teaspoons chopped capers

3 tablespoons (42 g) Good Ol' Mayonnaise (See page 30.)

¼ of a lemon, grated zest and juice

Per serving: 397 calories, 35 g fat, 22 g protein, 2 g carbohydrate, trace dietary fiber, 2 g net carbs

Sunshine Chicken Salad

SERVES 2

I was talking about my work with my dear friend Tonya and fancifully said, off the top of my head, "Or a chicken salad with grapefruit and white balsamic vinaigrette." After a moment's thought, I said, "Y'know, that sounds good." It is. It's perfect for a special lunch with friends!

If the chicken is cold, warm it up. (I gave mine just a minute on 70 percent power in the microwave.)

While that's happening, put the lettuce in a salad bowl.

Hold the grapefruit half over a bowl to catch the juice and use a small, thin-bladed knife to cut out the sections. Squeeze the juice out of the remains when all the sections are out.

Measure the dressing and add the grapefruit juice to it. Shake it up, pour it over the salad, and toss it to coat.

Pile the greens on two plates. Top each with half of the grapefruit sections, onion, and chicken. Serve immediately.

1 cup (140 g) diced cooked chicken

7 ounces (200 g) bagged salad (Get one with some radicchio and frisée if they have it.)

½ of a ruby red grapefruit

¼ cup (60 ml) White Balsamic Vinaigrette (See page 31.)

⅛ of a small red onion, sliced paper-thin

Per serving: 347 calories, 17 g fat, 37 g protein, 10 g carbohydrate, 3 g dietary fiber, 7 g net carbs

notes

I used the last of a chicken I'd roasted earlier in the week, warmed up, and it was great. If you have no cooked chicken on hand, a boneless, skinless chicken breast takes only 5 minutes or so in an electric contact grill and only a minute or two longer in a skillet.

I used bagged salad that included romaine and radicchio, along with some other lettuces and some shredded carrot. It was perfect for this, but I think the most important parts were the romaine and radicchio. Peruse the organic bagged salad selection at your grocery or health food store and see if you can find the two together.

You want a really juicy grapefruit! Weigh them in your hand: the heavier, the better. Thin-skinned is better than thick; they're juicier. Just squeeze gently to feel how much the skin gives.

Chicken, Orange, and Olive Salad

I first made this from the remains of a rotisserie chicken. Yummy! If you don't happen to have a rotisserie chicken on hand, it's a matter of 5 minutes to cook a boneless, skinless breast in an electric contact grill and maybe 7 to 8 minutes to sauté one.

Grate ½ teaspoon of zest from the orange. Now halve it and holding it over a bowl to catch the juice, use a small, sharp, thin-bladed knife to cut around the sections. Put the freed-up sections in another bowl as you go. When they're all cut out, squeeze the rest of the juice from the rinds into the juice bowl.

Add the zest and the juice to the vinaigrette and shake it up.

Pile the greens in a salad bowl. Pour on the now-orange-y vinaigrette and toss like mad till they're all evenly coated. Pile the greens on two plates. Top each salad with half of the chicken, olives, and orange sections and then serve.

SERVES 2

1 orange

½ cup (120 ml) White Balsamic Vinaigrette (See page 31.)

4 cups (220 g) spring mix greens

6 ounces (170 g) diced cooked chicken

12 Kalamata olives, pitted and chopped

Per serving: 547 calories, 41 g fat, 30 g protein, 16 g carbohydrate, 5 g dietary fiber, 11 g net carbs

Tuna Salad Vinaigrette

We've all grown up with tuna salad made with mayo, so I thought I'd throw it a curve. If you like, you could save a step and serve this stuffed into the hollow of a halved avocado.

In a mixing bowl, combine everything but the avocado and stir it together.

Peel, pit, and slice the avocado and fan the slices prettily on two plates. Top each with half of the tuna mixture and serve immediately.

SERVES 2

6 ounces (170 g) tuna in olive oil

¼ cup (40 g) diced red onion

2 tablespoons (2 g) minced cilantro

⅓ cup (80 ml) vinaigrette (Balsamic Vinaigrette on page 31 or Italian Vinaigrette on page 32 will work nicely.)

1 avocado

Per serving: 525 calories, 43 g fat, 27 g protein, 10 g carbohydrate, 3 g dietary fiber, 7 g net carbs

Definitely Not Nicoise Salad

SERVES
4

Traditional Nicoise has potatoes, not radishes, and a whole bunch of other stuff. But once I tried boiling radishes, this seemed like a better and better idea. Yummy! And it's a great make-ahead.

Start by putting the radishes in a saucepan, covering them with water, and bringing them to a simmer. Let them cook for 30 minutes until tender. Drain and cool.

In the meantime, trim the green beans. Now you have a decision to make: Leave them whole—more picturesque—or cut 'em in halves or thirds—easier to handle. Either way, steam them for 12 minutes until tender but not mushy. Put them in a mixing bowl.

Are your radishes cool? Good. Slice 'em into rounds. Throw them in with the beans. Pour on the vinaigrette and stir it up.

Open the can of tuna. You don't want to drain it really thoroughly, just pour off what oil pours off easily. Dump the tuna into the salad and mix it up gently, leaving some big hunks of tuna. Chill the whole thing. When the time comes to serve it, pile it on plates (or in bowls, what do I care?). Peel and slice the hard boiled eggs and top each serving with the pretty white-and-yellow rounds.

8 ounces (225 g) trimmed radishes

12 ounces (340 g) green beans

⅓ cup (80 ml) White Balsamic Vinaigrette (See page 31.)

10 ounces (280 g) tuna packed in olive oil

4 eggs, hard-boiled

Per serving: 285 calories, 17 g fat, 24 g protein, 8 g carbohydrate, 3 g dietary fiber, 5 g net carbs

note

If I were going to add anything to this—not that it needs anything, because it doesn't—I'd go with halved grape or cherry tomatoes. They'd both taste good and look pretty.

Simple Crab Salad

Butter lettuce to wrap this salad in would be nice, but you could always use a fork.

It's pretty simple: Put the crab meat in a mixing bowl and throw in the celery.

In another bowl, mix together the mayonnaise, sour cream, and dill. Pour it over the crab and celery and mix.

Season the salad with salt and pepper and serve immediately.

1 pound (455 g) lump crabmeat

½ cup (50 g) chopped celery

½ cup (115 g) Good Ol' Mayonnaise (See page 30.)

¼ cup (60 g) Coconut Sour Cream (See page 37.)

1 tablespoon (4 g) minced fresh dill weed

Salt and ground black pepper, to taste

Per serving: 329 calories, 28 g fat, 21 g protein, 1 g carbohydrate, trace dietary fiber, 1 g net carbs

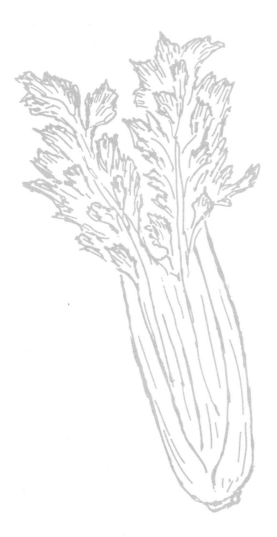

Roasted Asparagus Salad with Poached Eggs

SERVES
4

This classic salad suits our needs perfectly. It's a great choice in early spring, when both asparagus and eggs go on sale.

Preheat the oven to 450°F (230°C or gas mark 8).

Snap the ends off the asparagus where they want to break naturally. Whack them into about 2 inch (5 cm) lengths. Lay them on your shallow roasting pan, toss with the oil to coat, and season with salt and pepper. Roast the asparagus for 10 to 15 minutes, depending on how thick the asparagus is, stirring once or twice. (You want it tender, with brown spots.) When the asparagus is done, remove it from the oven and let it cool. (You can do this part in advance, if you like.)

When mealtime approaches, put about 2 inches (5 cm) of water in a skillet. (Yes, a skillet.) Add a little salt. If you're willing to go with 1 more ingredient, add 1 tablespoon (15 ml) of vinegar, but it's not essential. Bring the water to a simmer.

In the meantime, break the eggs into four custard or coffee cups. Slip 'em into the water very gently, turn off the heat, cover the skillet, and let the residual heat cook them. (You want the whites set, but the yolks till runny.)

While the eggs are poaching, grab the asparagus and toss in a bowl with ¼ cup (60 ml) of the dressing.

Dump the arugula in a salad bowl, pour on the rest of the dressing, and toss that, too. Pile the arugula on four plates. Top each with one-quarter of the asparagus, then 2 poached eggs. On top of each, scatter 2 tablespoons (10 g) of the Parmesan cheese and serve immediately.

2 pounds (900 g) asparagus

3 tablespoons (45 ml) olive oil

Salt and ground black pepper, to taste

8 eggs

8 ounces (225 g) arugula

½ cup (120 ml) White Balsamic Vinaigrette (see page 31), divided

½ cup (40 g) shredded Parmesan cheese

Per serving: 407 calories, 34 g fat, 18 g protein, 9 g carbohydrate, 3 g dietary fiber, 6 g net carbs

Beverages

The most Paleo of beverages is, of course, water. If you're a water drinker, have at it. It's good stuff. That said, the idea that all beverages are nutritionally inferior to water is simply untrue.

Tea and coffee both add antioxidants, as does the hibiscus in the Ruby Relaxer on page 164. Lemon adds vitamins; coconut milk adds immune-bolstering, thyroid-stimulating coconut oil. Heavy cream, especially from grass-fed cows, adds vitamin A of the best kind, as well as cancer-suppressing, belly-fat-burning CLA. So drink up to your good health.

Lemonade

I wanted to include this simple recipe so you will be able to make Angelia's Strawberry Arnold Palmers on page 162. Tester Rebecca says everyone loved it and that comparing the taste to ease and quickness of preparation she'd give this a perfect 10.

Mix everything in a half-gallon (1.9 L) pitcher and chill well. Serve over ice.

SERVES 8

1¼ cups (285 ml) fresh lemon juice

½ teaspoon lemon zest

1 teaspoon lemon–flavored liquid stevia extract, or to taste

7 cups (1.6 L) water

Per serving: 10 calories, trace fat, trace protein, 3 g carbohydrate, 0 g dietary fiber, 3 g net carbs

Strawberry Iced Tea

Tester Rebecca says that unless you can get really ripe, in-season strawberries, you might want to go with frozen. They'll be more flavorful than off-season fresh strawberries. Thaw them first, or they'll cool the tea too quickly, and pour in all the juice from the bag.

Put the tea bags, stevia, and strawberries in a ½-gallon (1.9 L) pitcher. Fill the pitcher with boiling water. Let it steep till it's cool.

Strain the tea, squeezing out the teabags to get all of the flavor, and return the tea to the pitcher. Add water to fill the space that used to be taken up by the strawberries. Chill the tea and serve over ice.

SERVES 8

8 tea bags, regular, decaf, or a mixture, as you prefer

¼ teaspoon plain or lemon–flavored liquid stevia extract, or to taste

1 pint (340 g) fresh strawberries, or, in a pinch, frozen without sugar

---

Per serving: 16 calories, trace fat, trace protein, 4 g carbohydrate, 1 g dietary fiber, 3 g net carbs

Angelia's Strawberry Arnold Palmers

SERVES 16

1 pitcher of Lemonade (See page 161.)

1 pitcher of Strawberry Iced Tea (See page 161.)

Per serving: 15 calories, trace fat, trace protein, 4 g carbohydrate, 1 g dietary fiber, 3 g net carbs

Credit for this idea goes to my friend and thrift-shopping buddy Angelia. We had stopped for lunch while doing our thrift-shopping rounds, and she ordered strawberry iced tea. Sipping it, she thoughtfully asked, "What about Strawberry Arnold Palmers?" I knew I had to do it.

Obviously, this requires you to make both Lemonade (see page 161) and Strawberry Iced Tea (see page 161). But because the Lemonade technically calls for only two ingredients not counting water—lemons and stevia—and the Strawberry Iced Tea calls for three—tea, strawberries, and stevia—this is still a five-ingredient recipe! Have both beverages made and chilled and simply mix them 50/50 over ice. If you have a 1-gallon (3.8 L) pitcher, you can mix both batches and have them on hand for guests. How perfect for a cookout!

Mix the Lemonade and Strawberry Iced Tea together over ice.

Coco-Caramel Coffee

SERVES 1

¾ cup (175 ml) hot, strong brewed coffee

¼ cup (60 ml) unsweetened coconut milk, warmed

12 drops of English toffee–flavored liquid stevia extract

Per serving: 114 calories, 12 g fat, 1 g protein, 2 g carbohydrate, 0 g dietary fiber, 2 g net carbs

You know that coffee "creamer" is among the most evil substances posing as food in your grocery store, right? This is so much better and so much better for you. Also, it's a snap to make.

Just put everything in a blender, run it for 15 seconds or so, pour, and drink. You can easily double or triple this if you've got more than one coffee drinker on hand.

Pumpkin Spice Colatte

You know how it is in the autumn: Suddenly pumpkin-spiced everything appears, including pumpkin-spiced lattes. Sadly, the stuff at coffee shops is full of sugar, and the flavored "creamers" at the grocery store are even worse. Quick, easy, and junk-free, this will fulfill all of your pumpkin-spice cravings.

Warm the coconut milk first, unless you want lukewarm coffee! Then just put everything in your blender and run it for a minute, until frothy. Pour the mixture into a mug and serve immediately.

 SERVES 1

½ cup (120 ml) coconut milk

½ cup (120 ml) strong, hot brewed coffee

1 teaspoon canned pumpkin

⅛ teaspoon English toffee–flavored stevia extract

⅛ teaspoon pumpkin pie spice

Per serving: 227 calories, 24 g fat, 2 g protein, 4 g carbohydrate, trace dietary fiber, 4 g net carbs

Peppermint Mocha

Watching television one Sunday morning, I saw an ad for "holiday creamers." Creamer is revolting stuff, a true chemical garbage-storm. But the flavors sounded easy to reproduce. Have this while you decorate the Christmas tree!

Just stir all of the ingredients together in a mug or run them through your blender.

 SERVES 1

¾ cup (180 ml) hot brewed coffee

¼ cup (60 ml) heavy cream or coconut milk, warmed

14 drops of dark chocolate–flavored liquid stevia extract

3 drops of peppermint extract

Per serving: 209 calories, 22 g fat, 1 g protein, 2 g carbohydrate, 0 g dietary fiber, 2 g net carbs

Ruby Relaxer

SERVES
8

Most of these herbs should be available at your health food store. Dried hibiscus flowers are available in Latin markets, in places with great bulk tea sections or, of course, online. I order from Mountain Rose herbs, www.mountainroseherbs.com.

Put all of the herbs into a ½-gallon (1.9 L) pitcher and pour boiling water over them to fill. Let the tea stand and brew till cool.

Strain the tea, pressing all you can out of the herbs, and then pour a little more water through the herbs to rinse all of the goodness out of them. Put the tea back in the pitcher and add water to fill. (Remember, some of the space in the pitcher during brewing will have been taken up by the herbs.) Chill the tea.

This makes a concentrate. I like to mix it about 50/50 with cold water or cold sparkling water, but dilute to taste.

1½ cups (45 g) dried hibiscus flowers

⅓ cup (6 g) dried lemon balm

⅓ cup (10 g) dried passion flower

2 tablespoons (8 g) orange peel

3 tablespoons (9 g) dried stevia herb, or to taste

Per serving: 1 calorie, trace fat, trace protein, trace carbohydrate, trace dietary fiber, 0 g net carbs

Sandman Sipper

SERVES
1

Want something comforting and relaxing before bed? This is perfect. If you're a caramel fiend, amplify the caramel flavor with the English toffee-flavored stevia. If you like caramel and chocolate, go with the chocolate-flavored stevia.

You can figure this out, right? Put the bag in a cup. Pour the water over it and let it steep for 5 minutes. Squeeze the bag as you remove it from the cup to get all of the flavor. Stir in the stevia and coconut milk and sip, preferably in front of a crackling fireplace or in a hot bath.

1 tea bag Yogi Caramel Bedtime Tea (You can find this at health food stores.)

6 ounces (175 ml) boiling water

12 drops of liquid stevia, chocolate–, English toffee–, or vanilla-flavored

3 tablespoons (45 ml) unsweetened coconut milk

Per serving: 89 calories, 9 g fat, 1 g protein, 2 g carbohydrate, trace dietary fiber, 2 g net carbs

Mocha-Nut Slush

Perfect for a hot summer morning, this requires that you have frozen coffee cubes. They're easy enough to make: Pour brewed, cooled coffee into ice cube trays and freeze it. Pop out the cubes, store them in a plastic bag, and you can make this in no time.

Put the coconut milk, chocolate extract, stevia, and vanilla extracts in your blender and turn it on. Remove the knob from the top and add the coffee ice cubes one at a time, letting each one get pulverized before you add the next. When they're all worked in, pour/spoon into a glass and eat!

SERVES
1

½ cup (120 ml) unsweetened coconut milk

¼ teaspoon natural chocolate extract

18 drops of chocolate-flavored liquid stevia extract, or to taste

¼ teaspoon vanilla extract

½ cup (120 ml) coffee, frozen in cubes

Per serving: 227 calories, 24 g fat, 2 g protein, 4 g carbohydrate, 0 g dietary fiber, 4 g net carbs

Coco-Cocoa

Tester Hanftka says, "The portions are generous for such a rich drink. But as Mae West is reputed to have said, 'Too much of a good thing is terrific.'"

You'll notice from the ingredients list that this is a can of coconut milk and a can of water, so rinse out the can to get the last bit of coconut milk. Put this in a heavy-bottomed saucepan over medium-low heat, along with everything else, and whisk until all of the cocoa is worked in. Bring the mixture to a simmer and serve immediately.

SERVES
3

1 can (14 ounces, or 410 ml) unsweetened coconut milk

1 can (14 ounces, or 410 ml) water

¼ cup (20 g) unsweetened cocoa

¼ teaspoon vanilla-flavored liquid stevia extract

1 pinch of salt

Per serving: 286 calories, 28 g fat, 4 g protein, 7 g carbohydrate, 2 g dietary fiber, 5 g net carbs

Coco-Mocha

Having tested the Coco-Cocoa, Hanftka suggested this terrific variation. What a great way to start a cold winter day!

You'll notice from the ingredients list that this is a can of coconut milk and a can of water, so rinse out the can. Put this in a heavy-bottomed saucepan over medium-low heat, along with everything else, and whisk until all the cocoa is worked in. Bring the mixture to a simmer and serve immediately.

SERVES
3

1 can (14 ounces, or 390 ml) unsweetened coconut milk

14 ounces (390 ml) brewed coffee

¼ cup (20 g) unsweetened cocoa

¼ teaspoon vanilla-flavored liquid stevia extract

¼ teaspoon cinnamon

1 pinch of salt

Per serving: 290 calories, 28 g fat, 4 g protein, 8 g carbohydrate, 2 g dietary fiber, 6 g net carbs

Soln Margarita

Dave Asprey, the Bulletproof Executive, has popularized the NorCal Margarita, vodka or tequila with a squeeze of lime, topped with club soda. This is how I make mine here in Southern Indiana.

Pour the tequila over a handful of ice cubes in a rocks glass. Squeeze in the lime juice and drop the wedge in the glass. Add the stevia and fill with the orange sparkling water.

SERVES
1

1 shot of tequila

Ice

1 wedge of lime

3 drops of plain or lemon-flavored liquid stevia extract

Orange-flavored sparkling water, chilled

Per serving: 69 calories, trace fat, trace protein, 2 g carbohydrate, trace dietary fiber, 2 g net carbs

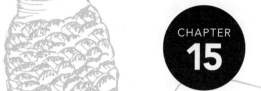

Sauces, Seasonings, and Condiments

Over the past couple of decades, there has been an explosion in the variety of condiments and seasonings available in the average grocery store. It's no mystery why: They give people a simple way to vary foods.

Keep your eyes open for garbage-free seasoning blends because they will make your life easier and more interesting.

Here you will find a variety of seasonings and sauces that will make your life more flavorful, without adding any sugar, cheap oils, or artificial flavors. Why aren't these in the Paleo Staples chapter? They struck me as being less staples and more for fun, for a change. I hope you like them!

Magic Dust

This is simply an all-natural flavor enhancer. You can use it in place of salt in just about any savory recipe, to good effect, though you'll want to increase the quantity. Use about twice as much of this as salt.

With the S-blade in place, run the mushrooms through a food processor until they're powdered. (This makes a fair quantity of fine dust that actually drifts out of the processor; I generally have to sweep a bit off the counter with my hand and put it back in. Be persistant.)

When the mushrooms are powdered, add the kelp and salt and run the food processor long enough to mix everything well. That's it! Put it in a spice shaker and keep it by the stove.

SERVES 8

2 ounces (28 g) dried shiitake mushrooms

1 tablespoon (5 g) kelp, powdered

¼ cup (135 g) sea salt

Per serving: 21 calories, trace fat, 1 g protein, 5 g carbohydrate, 1 g dietary fiber, 4 g net carbs

Shortcut Mole

I used Lily's brand stevia-sweetened chocolate chips, but I confess that, owing to a touch of soy lecithin, they cannot be considered truly Paleo-kosher. For my purposes, the lack of sugar was more important. Many Paleo folks have a favorite brand of dark chocolate they consider acceptable. If you do, I'm sure it will be fine here, though depending on how dark it is, you may want to add a little stevia or honey. You could also use bitter baking chocolate—1½ ounces (43 g)—plus honey or stevia.

Just put the salsa in a saucepan and bring it to a simmer. Whisk in the chocolate and cinnamon, stirring until the chocolate melts. That's it.

SERVES 6

2 cups (520 g) chipotle salsa

2 ounces (55 g) semisweet chocolate (Use your favorite Paleo chocolate.)

½ teaspoon cinnamon

Per serving: 70 calories, 3 g fat, 1 g protein, 12 g carbohydrate, 1 g dietary fiber, 11 g net carbs

Hot 'n Fruity Barbecue Sauce

SERVES
12

Commercial barbecue sauce is very sugary, even more so than ketchup. For those of you who have to keep your carbs low, note that sugar from fruit is sugar all the same. Still, this has considerably less sugar than the commercial stuff.

In a nonreactive saucepan—stainless steel, enamel, or stove-top compatible glass—combine the salsa and water. Add the prunes, bring to a low simmer, and let it cook for 10 to 15 minutes.

Use a stick blender to puree the whole thing or dump it in your blender and run it till it's smooth. Grate in the zest from the orange half, and then squeeze in all of the juice. Blend in the chili powder and stevia.

If you're using a regular blender, pour the sauce back into the pan and put it back over low heat. Let it simmer for another 10 minutes to let the flavors blend. When cooled, pour it into the salsa jar to store.

1 jar (16 ounces, or 455 g) salsa

½ cup (120 ml) water

4 prunes

½ of an orange

1 tablespoon (8 g) chili powder

⅛ teaspoon English toffee–flavored liquid stevia extract

Per serving: 22 calories, trace fat, 1 g protein, 5 g carbohydrate, 1 g dietary fiber, 4 g net carbs

Not Peanut Sauce

SERVES
4

Thai peanut sauce is very popular, but, being legumes, peanuts aren't Paleo. Further, real peanut sauce calls for a whole slew of ingredients. This is utterly inauthentic, but it's fast, easy, and good anywhere you'd use peanut sauce. Serve it with chicken, pork, or shrimp—anything, really.

Just run everything through your blender or food processor.

1⅓ cups (347 g) salsa

¼ cup (65 g) almond butter

4 teaspoons (20 ml) fish sauce

Per serving: 126 calories, 9 g fat, 5 g protein, 9 g carbohydrate, 3 g dietary fiber, 6 g net carbs

Korean-ish Seasoning Sauce

Korean cooking tends to seasoning with lots of soy sauce and sugar. Here, coconut aminos stand in for the soy sauce, and honey subs for the sugar. If you're going to add anything to this, I'd go with a shot of sriracha.

Just stir everything together. That's it!

½ cup (120 ml) coconut aminos

2 teaspoons honey

2 teaspoons dark sesame oil

Per serving: 30 calories, 1 g fat, trace protein, 4 g carbohydrate, trace dietary fiber, 4 g net carbs

Bacon-Mayo

I'd call it Baconnaise, but that name is trademarked. I have no idea if this is even close to the original because the original is a perfect storm of Garbage I Won't Eat. This is awfully good, regardless.

Put the egg yolk, stevia, and Creole Seasoning in a food processor.

In a glass measuring cup, measure and stir together the bacon grease and oil.

Turn on the food processor and while it's running, slowly pour in the bacon grease/oil mixture. (You want a stream about the diameter of a pencil lead.) When it's all in, turn off the food processor.

My Bacon-Mayo was still pourable at this point, but I knew that, owing to the bacon grease, it would thicken with refrigeration, and it did. So don't panic when your Bacon-Mayo is too runny when you finish processing. It'll be fine after chilling.

1 egg yolk

Liquid stevia extract to equal ½ teaspoon sugar

1 tablespoon (11 g) Creole Seasoning (See page 35.)

½ cup (112 g) bacon grease

½ cup (120 ml) MCT oil or light olive oil

Per serving: 129 calories, 14 g fat, trace protein, 1 g carbohydrate, trace dietary fiber, 1 g net carbs

Bacon Jazz

SERVES
8

This started with Bacon Jam by the Domestic Diva. It sounded great, but it had too many ingredients and way too much sugar (in the form of maple syrup) for my tastes. So I played with the idea and came up with this. It's fab! Try it on a burger, mix it into veggies, or whatever.

Lay the bacon across your cutting board and cut it into ½-inch (1.3 cm) lengths. Put a big, heavy skillet over medium-low heat, throw in the bacon, and start it browning.

In the meantime, peel and chop the onion, taking·a moment now and then to stir the bacon.

When the bacon bits are crisp—watch for foaming, a sign they're getting close—scoop out the bacon bits with a slotted spoon to a plate and reserve.

Pour off all but a few tablespoons (45 to 60 ml) of fat. Put the skillet back over the burner and turn the heat to low. Add the onion, stir it up, and then spread it out. (You're going to cara-melize it. This is going to take a few minutes, so pour yourself a cup of tea.)

Stir the bacon bits back in and add the maple syrup or other sweetener, mustard, and water. Stir them in till everything is very well acquainted. Let it all cook for another 5 minutes, stirring now and then, and proclaim it good!

1 pound (455 g) bacon

1 red onion

3 tablespoons (60 g) maple syrup or (36 g) erythritol plus ⅛ teaspoon maple extract

2 tablespoons (30 g) spicy brown mustard

2 teaspoons water

Per serving: 357 calories, 28 g fat, 18 g protein, 7 g carbohydrate, trace dietary fiber, 7 g net carbs

Apricot Sauce and Glaze

SERVES 6

With vinegar, mustard, ginger, and garlic, this fruity sauce bears a resemblance to chutney. Try it with chicken brushed with butter melted with curry powder! You can serve this simply spooned over chicken or pork. To use it as a glaze, you'll want to thin it a bit with water.

Put the apricots in a small nonreactive saucepan. Add the water and bring it to a low simmer. Cover the pan and let the apricots simmer till soft.

Dump the apricots and water in your food processor and add the vinaigrette, ginger, and mustard. Run till the apricots are pretty much pulverized and you have a thick sauce.

2 ounces (55 g) dried apricot halves

½ cup (120 ml) water

½ cup (120 ml) White Balsamic Vinaigrette (See page 31.)

2 teaspoons grated ginger root

1 teaspoon spicy brown mustard

Per serving: 117 calories, 11 g fat, trace protein, 7 g carbohydrate, 1 g dietary fiber, 6 g net carbs

note

Mixed 50/50 with mayonnaise, this is wonderful on chicken salad.

Apricot Dipping Sauce

SERVES 4

If you've made the Apricot Sauce and Glaze above, this is an easy and obvious way to use it. It's great on chicken salad or as a dipping sauce for Chicken Nuggets (see page 66). You'll note that—assuming mayonnaise counts as a staple—this is only five ingredients.

Just stir 'em together. That's it.

½ cup (120 ml) Apricot Sauce and Glaze (See recipe above.)

½ cup (115 g) Good Ol' Mayonnaise (See page 30.)

Per serving: 256 calories, 29 g fat, 1 g protein, 3 g carbohydrate, trace dietary fiber, 3 g net carbs

White Butter Sauce

A riff on beurre blanc, a traditional French sauce, this is rich and delicious. This will make any simple white fish very special. I served it to my husband over cod, and he licked the plate.

In a small, nonreactive saucepan over medium-low heat, combine the wine and shallot. Bring the mixture to a simmer and cook it till the wine is reduced to about 1 tablespoon (15 ml).

In the meantime, cut the butter into tablespoon (14 g) pats, and then quarter each of those.

When the wine is reduced, grab a stick blender. Start blending the wine mixture as you add one little lump of butter at a time, letting it melt completely before you add another. Your sauce should thicken and emulsify a bit, becoming creamy.

When all of the butter is in, it's done!

SERVES 2

¼ cup (60 ml) dry white wine

½ of a shallot, minced, about two teaspoons

3 tablespoons (42 g) butter

Per serving: 174 calories, 17 g fat, trace protein, 1 g carbohydrate, 0 g dietary fiber, 1 g net carbs

note

You can make this with chilled ghee if you like, adding a teaspoon at a time till you've incorporated 3 tablespoons (45 ml) worth (9 teaspoons). But don't bother trying it with oil. It's better to go with a different recipe altogether.

White Wine Sauce

I first created this for steamed mussels, but try it with scallops, shrimp, or even a simple fish fillet.

In a saucepan over medium-low heat, melt the butter. Throw in the shallots and sauté them until they're starting to soften. Add the wine and the fennel seed and bring to just below a simmer. Let the whole thing cook for 6 to 7 minutes until it's reduced a little.

SERVES 4

1 stick of butter

4 shallots, finely minced

1 cup (235 ml) dry white wine

1 teaspoon ground fennel seed

Per serving: 252 calories, 23 g fat, 1 g protein, 2 g carbohydrate, trace dietary fiber, 2 g net carbs

Desserts

The easiest and most Paleo dessert is fresh fruit, whatever is in season. If you're feeling ambitious, you can add cream, plain or whipped, to berries, a drizzle of yacon syrup (see page 18) or honey to half a grapefruit, or gild the lily in some other way.

If you're downright frisky, you could make fruit salad. Just cut up any three or four fruits in season and combine. Primal folks can stir a little vanilla-flavored liquid stevia extract into plain Greek yogurt and add sliced berries. Sprinkle with Coconut Maple-Cinnamon Flakes (see page 51) or chopped nuts, and you have a sundae.

Beyond that? As mentioned in the Introduction, eating sweets in quantity, or regularly, is of questionable Paleo authenticity, regardless of the ingredients. The higher carb of these recipes can really only be recommended for people who are naturally slender and athletic. There are, however, desserts in this chapter low carb enough even for Atkins Induction. Just pay attention to the nutritional stats, okay?

Jungle Bars

Dried bananas are not the same thing as banana chips, but rather the banana equivalent of a raisin or prune. Order them online if you can't find them locally.

Preheat the oven to 350°F (180°C or gas mark 4). Grease an 8- × 8-inch (20 × 20 cm) baking pan.

Chop the dried bananas into pieces about the size of a raisin. Transfer to a food processor.

Add the coconut and salt. Process until the bananas and coconut are pretty well incorporated—with just flecks of banana left. Add the egg and stevia and run just until well blended.

Turn the dough out into the prepared pan and use the back of a spoon to press it out firmly into an even layer. Bake for 20 to 25 minutes or until getting golden just around the edges. Cool, cut into bars, and store in a snap-top container.

SERVES 16

1 cup (224 g) dried bananas

2 cups (160 g) shredded coconut

¼ teaspoon salt

1 egg

¼ teaspoon vanilla-flavored liquid stevia extract

Per serving: 64 calories, 4 g fat, 1 g protein, 8 g carbohydrate, 2 g dietary fiber, 6 g net carbs

Apple-Walnut Bars

These are great with a cup of coffee or tea. Store in the fridge! These will go moldy kept at room temperature.

Preheat the oven to 350°F (180°C or gas mark 4). Grease an 8- × 8-inch (20 × 20 cm) baking pan.

Quarter and core the apple. Cut the quarters in half again. Throw 'em in a food processor with the walnuts, cinnamon, and salt. Pulse till everything is a medium-coarse consistency. Add the egg and the stevia and run again until everything is mixed, but don't over chop.

Turn the dough out into the prepared pan and use the back of a spoon to press it out into an even layer. Bake for 20 minutes. Cool and then cut in squares.

SERVES 16

1 apple

2 cups (200 g) walnuts

1 teaspoon cinnamon

¼ teaspoon salt

1 egg

¼ teaspoon English toffee–flavored liquid stevia extract

Per serving: 104 calories, 9 g fat, 4 g protein, 3 g carbohydrate, 1 g dietary fiber, 2 g net carbs

Notmeal Cookies

These are chewy and cinnamon-y. The count and nutritional stats assume you're making bite-sized cookies, not bigger ones.

Preheat the oven to 350°F (180°C or gas mark 4). Line a couple of cookie sheets with baking parchment.

Put all but ¼ cup (20 g) of the coconut in a food processor, with the S-blade in place. Add the salt and cinnamon and run until you have coconut butter. (This will take at least 10 minutes.)

Now add the honey and eggs and run it until you have a well-blended, sticky, soft dough. Add the flaxseed meal and the last ¼ cup (20 g) of coconut and pulse just until they're blended in.

Drop by teaspoonfuls onto the parchment paper and spread a tiny bit with the back of a spoon. Bake for 12 minutes, check for doneness, and give another 2 to 3 minutes if needed. Cool on a wire rack and store in a snap-top container.

SERVES 36

4½ cups (360 g) shredded coconut, divided

¼ teaspoon salt

1 teaspoon cinnamon

¼ cup (80 g) honey

2 eggs

½ cup (56 g) golden flaxseed meal

Per serving: 62 calories, 5 g fat, 1 g protein, 5 g carbohydrate, 2 g dietary fiber, 3 g net carbs

Almond Butter Cookies

The texture will depend on how finely ground your almond butter is. Mine is coarse, so I get chunks of nut in my cookies.

Preheat the oven to 350°F (180°C or gas mark 4). Line 2 cookie sheets with baking parchment or grease them well.

Using an electric mixer, beat the almond butter, egg, and salt together until thoroughly blended. Now beat in the sweeteners, all three of them, until the whole thing is evenly blended.

Using clean hands, form the dough into 1-inch (2.5 cm) balls and arrange them on the cookie sheets. Use a fork to flatten the balls, making crosshatch marks. Bake for 10 minutes. The cookies will be very soft, so let them cool on the sheets for at least 10 minutes before removing to a wire rack to finish cooling. Store in a snap-top container.

SERVES 20

1 cup (260 g) almond butter

1 egg

½ teaspoon salt (If your almond butter includes salt, you may not need this.)

½ cup (96 g) erythritol

¼ teaspoon vanilla-flavored liquid stevia extract

1 tablespoon (15 ml) yacon syrup (See page 18.)

Per serving: 79 calories, 7 g fat, 3 g protein, 2 g carbohydrate, 2 g dietary fiber, 0 g net carbs

Almond Meringues

Light, airy, crisp, and sweet, these meringues will please more than just the Paleo crew. They not only serve as cookies, but they make a great dessert topping.

Preheat the oven to 350°F (180°C or gas mark 4).

Spread the almonds in a shallow baking sheet and bake them for just 5 minutes. Remove them from the oven and turn the temperature down to 250°F (120°C or gas mark ½). Line two cookie sheets with baking parchment.

Put the almonds in a food processor. Pulse until they're chopped medium-fine, with the biggest bits about half the size of a pea.

Put the egg whites in a deep mixing bowl. Use an electric mixer, not a blender or food processor, at the highest speed and start whipping the whites. When they start to get foamy and expand in volume, add the salt. Now start adding the erythritol, sprinkling it in 1 tablespoon (12 g) at a time, making sure one is completely incorporated before you add another. By the time you finish adding the erythritol, the whites should be very stiff, mounding up around the beaters. Beat in the vanilla and then turn off the mixer.

Add all but about 3 tablespoons (27 g) of the chopped almonds to the egg white mixture. Use a rubber scraper to quickly and lightly fold them in.

Now scoop the meringue onto the cookie sheets. (I used a cookie scoop, which holds 2 tablespoons [28 g].) Sprinkle a pinch of the reserved almonds on each one.

Bake the meringues for 20 minutes at 250°F (120°C or gas mark ½). Turn the oven down to 200°F (93°C) and bake them for another 25 minutes. Now turn the oven down to 170°F (77°C). Dry for another 30 minutes.

Cool the meringues on cookie sheets before using a spatula to carefully remove from the parchment.

1 cup (145 g) almonds

5 egg whites

1 pinch of salt

½ cup (96 g) erythritol

1 teaspoon vanilla extract, almond extract, or ½ teaspoon of each

Per serving: 21 calories, 2 g fat, 1 g protein, 1 g carbohydrate, trace dietary fiber, 1 g net carbs

notes

For ideas to use up those extra yolks, see Egg Yolk Dip on page 42 or Chocolate Pudding Custard on page 179.

If you like, you can use this same mixture to make a pie shell. Just swirl it into a greased pie plate, building it up the sides, and bake as usual. Fill it with fruit, custard, whatever you like.

Almond Cake

SERVES
12

Moist, a little sticky, and super tasty, this is just the thing with a cup of coffee. This cake is all about technique. You really have to whip the eggs very well because they're your only leavening; it helps to have a stand mixer. You must incorporate the eggs into the almond butter gradually.

Preheat the oven to 350°F (180°C or gas mark 4). Line the bottom of a 9½-inch (24 cm) springform pan with nonstick foil and grease the sides. (You can go down to 9 inch (23 cm) or up to 10 inch (25 cm), but don't stray any further.)

Put the eggs in a deep, narrow bowl and whip them on high speed for 10 minutes. Yes, for 10 minutes. If you have a stand mixer, you can start measuring the rest of the stuff while the eggs whip.

In a saucepan over low heat, warm the almond butter and honey together and stir together very well. Whisk in the cinnamon, stevia, and salt. Remove from the burner. (You want this soft but not hot enough to cook the eggs.)

Okay, your eggs have been thoroughly whipped. Scoop about one-quarter of the eggs into the pan with the almond butter. Using a rubber scraper, fold the eggs into the almond butter mixture. Add another one-quarter of the eggs, and again, fold them in thoroughly. Repeat twice, with the remaining eggs, until they're all folded in. Scrape this mixture into your prepared springform pan.

Bake for 20 minutes and then check. If it's not pulling away from the sides of the pan, give it another 5 minutes and check again. (You're looking for that sign.)

Remove the cake from the oven and let it cool completely in the springform pan before removing the sides.

6 eggs

1 cup (260 g) almond butter

¼ cup (80 g) honey

1 teaspoon cinnamon

¼ teaspoon English toffee–flavored liquid stevia extract

¼ teaspoon salt

Per serving: 181 calories, 14 g fat, 7 g protein, 10 g carbohydrate, 3 g dietary fiber, 7 g net carbs

Chocolate Pudding Custard

SERVES 6

The first time I made this, I was disappointed that it didn't set up firm like a custard. But it was super yummy! Then I realized that while it didn't have the texture of a custard, it was a perfect pudding. Hooray!

Preheat the oven to 300°F (150°C or gas mark 2). Grease a glass baking dish, such as Pyrex.

Warm the chocolate and coconut milk together, either in a saucepan over low heat or in a microwave-safe bowl, for 5 minutes at 50 percent power in the microwave.

Pour the chocolate/coconut milk mixture into a blender and get it running. With the blender running, add the egg yolks, one by one. Now blend in the stevia and salt. Make sure the whole thing is smooth.

Place the greased baking dish in a baking pan just big enough to hold it. (I used an 8- × 8-inch [20 × 20 cm].) Pour the custard mixture into the baking dish. Pour the hottest tap water your sink produces into the pan outside the baking dish.

Put the whole thing in the oven. Bake for 1 hour. Turn off the oven and crack the door to let the heat out. Let it cool till you can handle the outside pan without getting scalded.

Remove the baking dish from the water, cover it with foil, and refrigerate overnight. Congratulations! You now have amazing chocolate pudding.

2 ounces (55 g) bitter baking chocolate

28 ounces (805 ml) unsweetened coconut milk

5 egg yolks

½ teaspoon liquid stevia (I used chocolate flavored, but vanilla would be good, too.)

Pinch of salt

Per serving: 358 calories, 37 g fat, 6 g protein, 6 g carbohydrate, 1 g dietary fiber, 5 g net carbs

Coconut-Almond Custard

This is rich and almost fudgy, with a slightly rough texture from the almond butter and a caramel flavor. It's the ultimate comfort food and great for breakfast! It'll keep you full for hours.

Preheat the oven to 300°F (150°C or gas mark 2). Grease a glass baking dish, such as Pyrex brand. Find a baking pan the dish fits into and set it in there.

This is a snap: Put everything into the blender and run it till the mixture is evenly blended. Pour it into the prepared baking dish.

Pour water into the surrounding pan, a good 1½ inches (3.8 cm) up the sides of the baking dish—but don't get water in the custard! Bake for 75 minutes and then cool and refrigerate before serving.

SERVES 6

1 can (14 ounces, or 410 ml) unsweetened coconut milk

½ cup (130 g) almond butter

¾ teaspoon English toffee–flavored liquid stevia extract

4 eggs

⅛ teaspoon salt

Per serving: 300 calories, 28 g fat, 9 g protein, 6 g carbohydrate, 3 g dietary fiber, 3 g net carbs

Energy Shots

These coffee jellies have both caffeine and medium chain triglycerides, making them the perfect snack when energy starts to flag. Plus they're a great way to work more gelatin into your diet.

Put the coffee in a blender and sprinkle the gelatin powder over it. Now turn on the blender and let it whomp that gelatin into the coffee. Add everything else and let it blend while you grease an 8- × 8-inch (20 × 20 cm) pan.

Turn off the blender, pour the coffee mixture into the pan, and stick it in the fridge. Let it chill for at least several hours, and overnight is great.

Cut the shots into 1-inch (2.5 cm) squares. Cover the pan with plastic wrap and keep refrigerated, though these will stand up to room temperature well enough to take several to work in a snap-top container.

SERVES 64

1 cup (235 ml) hot brewed coffee

5 tablespoons (35 g) unflavored gelatin

½ cup (120 ml) unsweetened coconut milk

2 tablespoons (28 ml) MCT oil

¼ teaspoon liquid stevia (I used vanilla flavored, but chocolate or English toffee would be great, too.)

Per serving: 12 calories, 1 g fat, trace protein, 1 g carbohydrate, 0 g dietary fiber, 1 g net carbs

Coffee Mousse

Creamy, rich, smooth, and fluffy, this dessert is suitable for company. It also makes a great summer breakfast, especially for you Bulletproof Coffee fans.

Put the gelatin in a small bowl and add the cold water. Let it sit for a few minutes till all the water has absorbed and the gelatin has swelled up. Now add the boiling water and stir till the gelatin dissolves.

In a medium-sized mixing bowl, combine the gelatin with the coffee, erythritol, stevia, and salt. Whisk till the erythritol is dissolved and everything is well combined. Put the bowl in the refrigerator and chill it till it's the texture of egg white.

When the gelatin mixture has thickened, you're ready to continue. Put the coconut milk in a small, deep mixing bowl and whip it on high until it's fluffy and thickened. (Don't expect it to turn out like whipped cream; it won't get that stiff.) Whip it for a good 4 to 5 minutes on high.

Grab the bowl of gelatin and use the same beaters to whip it till it, too, is fluffy and thickening.

Now, with the mixer running, add the coconut milk to the gelatin mixture. Whip them together. Now spoon/scrape into four pretty dessert dishes and chill them for at least several hours and overnight is great.

1½ teaspoons unflavored gelatin powder

2 tablespoons (28 ml) cold water

3 tablespoons (28 ml) boiling water

1 cup (235 ml) strong brewed coffee, regular or decaf, as you prefer

¼ cup (48 g) erythritol

¼ teaspoon liquid stevia (I used chocolate flavored, but vanilla or English toffee would be good here, too.)

Tiny pinch of salt

1 can (14 ounces, or 410 ml) unsweetened coconut milk, chilled

---

Per serving: 5 calories, trace fat, 1 g protein, trace carbohydrate, 0 g dietary fiber, trace net carbs

note

If you're willing to take the trouble —and the extra ingredient—to garnish this, a little cocoa powder or espresso-grind coffee dusted on top looks pretty and tastes good.

Cacao Nib Frozen Custard

Cacao nibs are bits of broken-up cacao beans, chocolate in its rawest form, and a good source of antioxidants. Health food stores carry them. You'll need an ice cream freezer for this.

In a large, heavy saucepan over very low heat, combine the coconut milk, vanilla, and cacao nibs. Bring the mixture very slowly to a simmer. (Mine took more than ½ hour to hit the simmering point.) Cover the pan, turn off the burner, and let it sit till it's lukewarm. (Don't skip this! A lot of this recipe is in the steeping of the ingredients, so the flavors can blend.)

In the meantime, separate the eggs, saving the whites for some other purpose—may I suggest meringues? Put the yolks in a good-sized heat-resistant bowl.

Okay, turn the burner back on, once again to low. Whisk the egg yolks together really well while the coconut milk is warming.

When the coconut milk is starting to get warm, use a ladle to transfer about ½ cup (120 ml) of it (the size of most ladles) to the bowl of yolks. Whisk this in well. Now transfer another ladleful of coconut milk to the bowl of yolks and again, whisk it in very well. Do this one more time, with a third ladleful of yolks.

Now you can pour the whole yolk mixture into the pan of coconut milk. Whisk in the salt and honey.

Stir constantly over low heat until the mixture thickens enough that it will coat a spoon and running a finger through that coating leaves a clean line. Congratulations! You have custard.

Refrigerate the custard overnight. No, really. I know, I know, you can barely stand it, but again, allowing time for flavors to steep and blend is essential.

Before you freeze the custard, strain it to remove the cacao nibs. Then pour the chilled custard into your ice cream freezer and freeze according to the directions that come with your unit.

2 cans (28 ounces, or 785 ml) unsweetened coconut milk

2 teaspoons vanilla extract

½ cup (64 g) cacao nibs

5 egg yolks

1 pinch of salt

⅓ cup (107 g) honey

Per serving: 370 calories, 32 g fat, 5 g protein, 20 g carbohydrate, trace dietary fiber, 20 g net carbs

notes

If you want to reduce the carb content of this recipe, add ¼ teaspoon vanilla-flavored liquid stevia extract and reduce the honey to 3 tablespoons (60 g).

I have no way to calculate the carbohydrate content added by the cacao nibs because the bulk of them are strained out. The 20 grams per serving comes from the coconut milk and honey.

Frozen Banana Bites

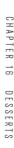

These are definitely not for the low-carb set, but they are a great treat for active kids on a hot summer afternoon.

In a bowl, combine the almond butter, coconut milk, and stevia thoroughly. (I'd use my little food processor because this wouldn't be enough stuff for a big one. If you only have a big one, work 'em together with a fork.)

Peel the bananas and cut them into bits about ¾ inch (2 cm) long.

It's assembly time! Lay a piece of waxed paper, nonstick foil, or baking parchment on a baking sheet. Sandwich banana slices together with the almond butter mixture, making a nice thick layer. Arrange them on the paper or foil. Put them in the freezer for an hour or so.

Put the chocolate in the top of a double boiler over hot water to start it melting. (My stove has a "simmer burner" that holds a steady temperature low enough for this job, but err on the side of caution. Chocolate scorches easily.)

When the chocolate is melted, pull the banana bites out of the freezer and spoon chocolate over each one, coating them as evenly as you can. If you like, you can spoon on one layer, chill them for another 10 minutes, and then spoon on a second layer.

Freeze 'em, pop them off of the paper or foil, and store them in a snap-top container in the freezer.

SERVES 8

⅓ cup (87 g) almond butter

2 tablespoons (28 ml) unsweetened coconut milk

¼ teaspoon vanilla- or coffee-flavored liquid stevia extract

2 bananas

3½ ounces (100 g) 85 percent dark chocolate

Per serving: 163 calories, 12 g fat, 4 g protein, 14 g carbohydrate, 4 g dietary fiber, 10 g net carbs

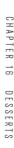

Sweet and Salty Pecans

This is a nice little nibble to pass in lieu of a big, set-piece dessert. Also these make great party food. You could even try them on a salad!

Preheat the oven to 350°F (180°C or gas mark 4). Line a shallow baking sheet with nonstick foil.

Put the egg white in a deep, narrow mixing bowl. With an electric mixer, start whipping the egg white. As it becomes frothy, sprinkle in 1 tablespoon (12 g) of the erythritol. As it becomes opaque and swells in volume, sprinkle in another tablespoon (12 g) and keep whipping.

When the egg white is stiff, turn off the mixer. With a rubber scraper, start stirring in the pecans, 1 cup (100 g) at a time, scraping all the way down to the bottom of the bowl. Work in all the pecans and make sure they're all evenly coated with the egg white mixture.

Spread the pecans on the foil in the baking sheet. Sprinkle evenly with ½ tablespoon (6 g) of the remaining erythritol and stir it in. Repeat with the rest of the erythritol. Now do the same with the salt, ½ teaspoon at a time. Spread the pecans in an even layer.

Slide 'em into the oven and set the timer for 5 minutes. When it beeps, stir them, spread them out again, and give them another 5 minutes. When the timer beeps again, stir them again, spread them out again, and put them back. Turn the oven down to 200°F (93°C). Set the timer for another 5 minutes.

When the timer beeps, stir and spread the pecans one last time. Put them back in and give them a final 10 minutes on that low temperature to make sure they're dried out and crispy. Pull 'em out, cool, and store in a snap-top container.

1 egg white, room temperature

3 tablespoons (36 g) erythritol, divided

4 cups (400 g) pecan halves

1 teaspoon salt

Per serving: 181 calories, 18 g fat, 2 g protein, 5 g carbohydrate, 2 g dietary fiber, 3 g net carbs

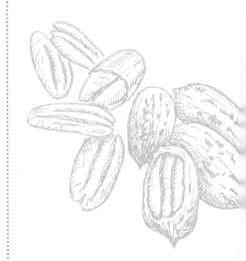

About the Author

In retrospect, Dana Carpender's career seems inevitable: She's been cooking since she had to stand on a step stool to reach the stove.

She was also a dangerously sugar-addicted child, eventually stealing from her parents to support her habit, and was in Weight Watchers by age eleven. At nineteen, Dana read her first book on nutrition, and she recognized herself in a list of symptoms of reactive hypoglycemia. She ditched sugar and white flour and was dazzled by the near instantaneous improvement in her physical and mental health. A lifetime nutrition buff was born.

Unfortunately, in the late 1980s and early 1990s, Dana got sucked into low-fat/high-carb mania, and whole-grain-and-beaned her way up to a size 20, with nasty energy swings, constant hunger, and borderline high blood pressure. In 1995, she read a nutrition book from the 1950s that stated that obesity had nothing to do with how much one ate, but was rather a carbohydrate intolerance disease. She thought, "What the heck, might as well give it a try." Three days later, her clothes were loose, her hunger was gone, and her energy level was through the roof. She never looked back, and she has now been low-carb for twenty years and counting—more than one-third of her life.

Realizing that this change was permanent, and being a cook at heart, Dana set about creating as varied and satisfying a cuisine as she could with a minimal carb load. And being an enthusiastic, gregarious sort, she started sharing her experience. By 1997, she was writing about it. The upshot is more than 2,500 recipes published and more than a million books sold—and she still has ideas left to try! Dana lives in Bloomington, Indiana, with her husband, three dogs, and a cat, all of whom are well and healthily fed.

Index